D0998326

DOCTOR, CAN YOU HEAR ME?

PATIENT, ARE YOU LISTENING?

DOCTOR, CAN YOU HEAR ME?

PATIENT, ARE YOU LISTENING?

MARGARET SMITH WASHINGTON, MSW, MSPH

with a foreword by **Thomas E. Starzl, MD, PhD**

Published by Washington Associates
http://www.doctorpatienttalk.com
8222 Rolfe Street, Pittsburgh, PA 15221
412-242-1964

ISBN 0-9747549-0-0
Printed in the United States of America.

Dedication

I dedicate this book to
Walter and Anna Mae Smith, my parents, who
encouraged me to spread my wings and fly;

Charles Edward Washington, my husband, who
encouraged me with love, support and understanding; and

Charles Michael, Sarah Michelle, and
Sharon Washington, my son, granddaughter,
and daughter-in-law, who make me smile.

Contents

Dr. Finikiotis, an internist at the University of Pittsburgh Medical Center (UPMC), believes that physicians' failure to communicate with patients compromises their ability to gather information, serves patients poorly, and adds to the cost of health care.

An editor and communications consultant to consumer and professional health care organizations, Ms. Albert offers some pointed advice to both groups for improving their communications and human relations skills.

An overview of the research conducted to document the extent to which doctors and patients are listening to and hearing each other and a preview to this book, which is based on the author's dialogue with more than 3,000 patients and physicians.

The responses of 2,400 patients and physicians to survey questions related to following instructions, physician availability, and the impact of regulatory agencies on patient care, aggregated by role (physician vs. patient) and analyzed by age, treatment setting, ethnicity, gender and time under physician care.

Pertinent and candid observations from the 375 individual patients who participated in focus groups on issues of communication, prescribing, and regulating, sampled and summarized numerically by category.

Acknowledgments

With much gratitude and humility, I acknowledge the support and cooperation of the chronically ill patients who allowed me to become part of their experience with candor and sensitivity. Among the many, Robert Franklin, Tyrone Oliver, Lawrence Washington (no relation to the author), Jane Mengel, and Rocco A. Duranti merit special mention.

I also acknowledge the many physicians who provided a learning experience for me, sharing both their great intellect and their humor. Although the number is large, a few must be publicly thanked for their support: Doctors Edward Barksdale, Susan Bray, Lawrence Ellis, Michael Finikiotis, Henri Ford, Robert Gerhardt, James Hanchett, Charles Hefflin, Derrick Latos, Velma Scantlebury, Charles Schleifer, Robert Sirota, Jeanette South-Paul, Thomas Starzl, and Mark Zeidel.

I am particularly grateful to my colleagues, Robert M. Grom, President and CEO, Heritage Health Foundation, and Margaret (Mimi) Priselac, President and CEO, UPMC Braddock, for their generous help in identifying funds to print this book.

Finally, my deep gratitude to my many friends who encouraged me when my dream of writing this book seemed impossible. Special thanks to Cynthia Jacobs, who taught me not to fear the dragon, to author and "wisewoman" M. Cecile Forte, PhD, who became my literary muse, and to Margaret (Peg) Albert, my friend and my editor, who put music to my words.

M.S.W.

Foreword

An Age-Old, Always New Adventure

No matter how well trained or how experienced we are as physicians, we are not delivering optimal care if we are not communicating with our patients. Learning is mutual when doctors and patients listen to and hear each other. Margaret Smith Washington reminds us of this. Moreover, she and her 3,000 physician and patient informants provide us with specific guidelines in her important book on how we can improve the lines of communication and, in the process, the quality of medical care.

The book is the culmination of three years of research by Washington, who is fully prepared academically and by hands-on experience to observe the ever-changing dynamics between doctors and patients. The author provides the reader with a snapshot of the many variables that affect the necessary dialogue between physicians and patients. Throughout, she illustrates the value of an equal partnership in ultimately reaching positive outcomes. The message is that if each party will listen to the other, both the patient and the doctor may accept new roles and responsibilities as a result of this age-old but always new adventure called improved communication.

The author has sounded an alarm and a call to action to address the crisis in communication. I recommend this book to practitioners as well as medical students and to patients and all those allied health professionals who guide them in finding the care they need.

Thomas E. Starzl, MD, PhD
Professor of Surgery
University of Pittsburgh Medical Center

Preface

A Practitioner's View

The practice of medicine has changed dramatically over the last decade. Advances in diagnosing and treating illnesses have been nothing short of amazing. At the same time, patient care has become increasingly technological and impersonal. Demands on doctors have grown more pressing and complex. Doctors must devote more time and attention to legal, insurance, and regulatory issues. The result is that many of them are spending less time with their patients.

Yet, even when doctors do take the time, they don't communicate effectively, according to many patients. These patients experience their doctors as distant and distracted. They complain that the doctors don't listen empathetically, frequently interrupting them before they've had a chance to finish speaking.

When doctors fail to communicate skillfully, their ability to gather information is compromised. They fail to engage patients in their own care and conduct or order unnecessary tests and treatments. All of this serves patients poorly and adds significant costs to health plans and plan sponsors.

In my practice, I find that patients want to be treated with humanity, dignity, and respect. Many seek detailed information that enables them to participate in making decisions about their treatment and care. Patients want and deserve the best care possible, and that entails receiving emotional and social support throughout their treatment process. Effective communication makes that possible.

The lion's share of responsibility for improving the dialogue with patients clearly rests with us as practitioners. Fortunately, the medical community is becoming sensitized to the virtues of effective communicating. Medical educators are adding communication courses to the basic curricula. Medical students are now learning skill-based patient interviewing techniques, though many patient advocates argue that such training must be greatly expanded in order to properly equip doctors in meeting their patients' needs.

Naturally, there are two sides to this equation. Patients, for their part, must become more participative in order to improve communications. In fact, research shows that patients who actively participate in their doctor visits realize better outcomes. Those who do take more responsibility in their care make better, more informed choices in receiving the support they need.

To that end, doctors can create a climate in which patients feel comfortable enough to participate more fully. For example, doctors can conclude patient visits with such questions as "Have I answered all your questions?" and "Is there anything else I can do for you?" Posing open-ended questions like these adds little time to the encounter but goes a long way toward encouraging more reticent patients to take an active role.

These are the issues that Margaret Smith Washington tackles in this book. In so doing, she seeks to restore the critical relationship between doctors and patients. She addresses the need for both parties to enter into full collaboration in order to improve the overall quality of health care.

She meticulously gathers the impressions of thousands of doctors and patients to present us with a convincing body of wisdom on the subject of communications. She opens our eyes to the perils of mutual misunderstanding and calls on both doctors and patients to approach the therapeutic relationship differently. Her prescription for both doctors and patients is clear and compelling: **Work together to eliminate barriers that hamper communication.**

To fulfill the promises of the last decade's impressive medical advances, doctors and patients must take definitive steps to improve their communication skills. *Doctor, Can You Hear Me? Patient, Are You Listening?* makes an irrefutable case for both to learn how to become partners in the process of patient care.

Michael W. Finikiotis, MD

Dr. Finikiotis is Board Certified in Internal Medicine. A private practitioner on the staff of the University of Pittsburgh Medical Center, he serves as Clinical Assistant Professor of Medicine in the University of Pittsburgh School of Medicine.

Preface

A Patient's View

C. Rufus Rorem, a pioneer in the voluntary pre-paid health insurance movement and an architect of the Blue Cross plans during the 1930s and '40s, had great respect for the patient. "I have often said that, in health care, man's best friend is himself," he wrote. "He is the one who is responsible for following the doctor's advice. Furthermore, a patient can be trusted, under supervision, to give himself tender and loving health care. He has no conflict of interest and nothing more important to do."

That simple statement (so typical in its clarity and substance of Rorem's superb capacity for communicating) is a challenge to both doctors and patients.

To physicians, it reiterates Sir William Osler's advice to "listen to the patient," and it quietly defies the common assumption that the non-compliant patient "doesn't care" about his health.

To patients, Rorem's statement is a call to become an active partner in our own health care and an expression of confidence in our ability to understand and follow the doctor's advice and to make choices that are in our own best interests.

As one who has interacted closely with physicians over the years in a professional capacity as a medical editor and writer, I have had access to the finest medical care available.

I've been cared for by physicians who respected my intelligence, my desire to learn, and my right to share in the decision-making, who welcomed my questions and took the time to help me understand fully what my options were and to keep me informed at all times, who cared deeply about me as a human being. For this experience, I shall be lastingly grateful. From this experience, I can relate easily to the spontaneous expressions of appreciation quoted in this book.

As the physicians I knew (and those who knew me) have retired or passed away, however, I have by default joined the ranks of common "referrals"—passed along impersonally to specialists on the basis of the condition of my lungs, my thyroid, or my uterus. Having become just another patient—and an aging one, at that—I find myself increasingly empathizing with the respondents in this book who complain that their physicians are condescending, impatient, and defensive. The care has been medically adequate in most cases, but the relationship and the level of communication often leave much to be desired.

In the preceding preface, Dr. Finikiotis (who appears to be the kind of doctor we all would like to have) lays the "lion's share of responsibility" for improving communication in the lap of the practitioner. In my view, it falls equally to doctor and patient, and I have some advice for both.

Doctor, I understand that you are practicing in the midst of constant change where the universe of scientific knowledge and the range of medications and technology are expanding by the hour and pressures from regulators are forcing you to do more for less and to do it more quickly. But that is not an excuse for the behaviors that are driving us apart.

I respect your expertise in medical science: that's why I ask questions. I expect you, in turn, to respect my intelligence and eagerness to learn more about my condition. I will follow your instructions when I can (and I am more likely to do so when I understand how the medication and/or lifestyle changes will improve my health.) What's more, in the face of today's information overload, an informed patient can be an effective partner in preventing medical errors.

I also expect you to respect my right to learn my test results promptly, my right to know the risks and benefits involved in any course of treatment, and—perhaps most difficult for you—my right to refuse treatment. This is where communication is most important. Discuss my reservations with me and, if possible, propose an alternative to simply walking away, but respect my right to reject your advice if that is my choice.

Fellow patient, you're not off the hook. Communication is a two-way street. If your physician doesn't tell you what you need or want to know, read everything you can find on the web and in the library about your condition. Jot down your questions, and present them on your next visit.

Have faith in your own knowledge about how you feel, what hurts, how much change in your lifestyle you and your family can tolerate, how much you can afford to pay for medications—and communicate these matters to your doctor. Physicians can assist you in finding help or alternative solutions when they are aware of the problem; they are unlikely to do so if they do not know a problem exists.

If your doctor refuses to listen to your concerns or resents answering your questions, look for a new doctor who will.

For more detailed suggestions for improving the lines of mutual communication between patients and physicians and for building the kind of partnership that is productive for both, I urge you to read the chapters that follow. From my years of association and friendship with the author, I know that she has seen doctor-patient interactions at their best and at their worst. She has done us all an immense favor by documenting the problem as well over 1,000 physicians and nearly 2,000 patients see it—and by providing invaluable suggestions for improving the clarity and substance of communication for all concerned. Rufus Rorem would have loved this book!

Margaret C. Albert

Ms. Albert, President of the Pittsburgh-based communications consulting firm, Matrix Communications Associates, has provided editorial services to medical publishers nationally and to several Pittsburgh hospitals and healthcare organizations as well as to the author of this book. She is a former managing editor of the Allegheny County Medical Society Bulletin and the author of A Practical Vision, the 50-year history of Blue Cross of Western Pennsylvania.

Introduction:
Hearing and Listening

The doctor says: ***"We're going to try a new medication for your blood pressure."*** *(Hands a prescription to the patient.)* ***"Get this filled today."***

The patient hears: ***"Another $60 at the pharmacy before my next check comes in."***

The patient says: ***"Let's wait a few weeks to start the new medicine."***

The doctor hears: ***"She's questioning my judgment. Why can't patients follow directions?"***

Too often, the exchanges between doctors and patients are like Alice's encounter with Humpty Dumpty in Lewis Carroll's *Through the Looking Glass.* When Humpty Dumpty used the word "glory" out of context, Alice told him, "I don't know what you mean by 'glory.'" Humpty Dumpty smiled contemptuously. "Of course you don't—till I tell you. . . . When I use a word, it means just what I choose it to mean—neither more nor less."[1]

Doctor-patient communication is often problematic. By definition and by connotation, words may have very different meanings to the doctor and to the patient. In addition to the complex language of medicine that can create a gulf in understanding, social and cultural factors can distance the physician from patients who live in a world he (or she) may never have visited. In the case of foreign-born physicians (or patients, for that matter), an accent or a limited understanding of idiomatic expressions may cause misunderstandings. Even more critical, perhaps, is the patient's failure to understand the seriousness of his or her condition and the need to comply with instructions and the physician's failure to understand the barriers—psychological, financial, or cultural—that may cause patient noncompliance.

Good communication is particularly important in the treatment of chronic illnesses such as hypertension, diabetes, and end-stage renal disease. Over the many years of interaction with physicians and their care teams, which include nurses, social workers, dietitians, and other health professionals, patients ideally develop a partnership with their physicians and care providers. Essential to this partnership is the commitment of both patient and physician to accomplish the best possible outcome. Patients must "own" their illness and the responsibility to follow medical direction, even when it means making significant life style changes. Both partners must pay particular heed to the art of "hearing and listening."

At no time has communication been more important than in today's health care system. Poor communication—an error in dosage, misunderstood instructions, or a failure to stress the importance of compliance—can lead to deadly errors, in the hospital and in the home. A May 2003

Medscape Instant Poll confirmed that communication was considered the major factor in non-pharmaceutical medical errors by 18 percent of physicians, 27 percent of medical students, 30 percent of pharmacists, and 16 percent of nurses. At the same time, however, the time that physicians can spend with patients is limited because of insurers' demands for greater productivity and economy, thus placing additional burdens on the communication process. There is little time for doctor and patient to "get to know each other," little time to repeat instructions, entertain questions, or expand upon concerns. Technological advances, which have brought such vast improvement to many aspects of medical care, including the electronic communication of data and information, have had no impact on the basic human interaction and communication between doctors and patients. Physicians continue to complain that patients "do not listen" while patients say doctors "do not hear me."

Doctor, Can You Hear Me? Patient, Are You Listening? is the product of more than three decades of first-hand observation in a variety of health care settings. In a neighborhood health center, in two major metropolitan teaching hospitals, and as Executive Director of a federally funded End-Stage Renal Disease Network of 160 dialysis facilities and 10 renal transplant centers, I saw the same kinds of poor communication: inattentiveness, misunderstanding, poor description of symptoms, equally poor explanation of diagnoses, rudeness, and cultural differences that became barriers to understanding. Finally, as a consultant on effective communication in health care, I am confronted regularly by patients and physicians who are looking for better ways to understand each other.

I determined to test my own observations by surveying 3,000 doctors and patients across the country, selected to reflect a diverse respondent pool geographically, culturally, and ethnically. Because of my close association with end-stage renal disease, I had initially planned to focus on this specific physician and patient group (nephrologists and transplant surgeons, dialysis and transplant patients). At the strong urging of the nephrologists with whom I spoke, however, I broadened the respondent group to include physicians and patients from diverse specialties such as family practice, internal medicine, surgery, oncology, obstetrics and gynecology, cardiology, pulmonary medicine, pediatrics, and endocrinology.

The brief surveys sent to physicians and patients asked about the problems they encountered and their ideas for improving doctor/patient communication. The response was overwhelming: nearly 80 percent of those who received the survey (2,392) completed it, and many physicians appended additional thoughts in attached notes or letters. To add depth and detail to the survey findings, I then embarked on a series of focus groups and individual interviews with a diverse population of nearly 700, including a professional football player, a medical director of a county health department, physician spouses of chronically ill patients, and others.

In all, more than 3,000 individuals—doctors, patients, and health professionals who were themselves patients—contributed to this book, creating a unique and intimate portrait of physician/patient interaction and the internal and external forces that impact on those relationships.

Across the board, more than one in four of both the physicians and the patients reported that the level of communication leaves much to be desired, and close to half of the patients found communication to be a serious problem. The respondents differed significantly by residence (rural *vs.* urban) and ethnicity in discussing their expectations and perceptions of care and of their roles as equal partners in the development of their treatment plans. Urban patients were more critical of health care providers in a number of areas, such as availability, office hours, costs, and frequency of prescription changes. Overall, rural patients were less likely to complain and, in the focus groups, more reticent in their responses. Similar differences emerged in comparing the racial groups: Caucasians were generally accepting of the care they received and reluctant to criticize their physicians while African Americans were more outspoken and often critical of the care, which, they perceived, was influenced by their race and ability to pay. The sampling of Hispanic and Asian patients was small, but they appeared most satisfied with their current health care delivery.

All of the physician participants were quite candid in their responses, but those who practiced in urban areas were more likely than their rural counterparts to expand upon their opinions, both in the surveys and in the focus groups. Not surprisingly, most physicians believed that they communicated much more effectively than the reports from the patient surveys and patient groups suggested. The breakdown in communication, according to the majority of the physicians, is the fault of "intrusive" government regulations, excessive paperwork requirements, and the "second-guessing" of insurance carriers that have interfered with their ability to practice and to relate effectively with their patients.

This diagnosis of the problem by a cross-section of the 21st century health care system is revealing in itself, but even more provocative is the incisive prescription for improving communication and, in the process, for improving the delivery of health care that emerges from their suggestions for change. As a result, this book speaks to a wide audience of patients and enlightened physicians and other health care professionals who understand that we are all, regardless of academic degree, social or economic status, patients at some point in our lives.

While I am certainly not the first to tackle the subject of doctor/patient communications, this book is unique in that it is, in a sense, a dialogue between doctors and patients in which the problems are identified and solutions are proposed. Whether the book is used as a text in medical school or continuing education courses, as a resource for in-service workshops or patient support groups, or simply as personal reading by patients or health professionals, it is my hope that its 3,000 voices will encourage readers to look within themselves for ways to bridge the gap between listening and hearing. The result can significantly improve not only their own level of communication but the overall quality of health care as well as we move toward a common language where even Alice and Humpty Dumpty may be able to agree on the meaning of words.

The Questionnaires
Surveying the Field

My doctor listens most of the time. I hear what he says sometimes.

(Patient)

HMOs direct patient care, no matter what anyone says. I have to compromise my standards of care to meet their requirements.

(Doctor)

The first step in testing the validity of my own view of communication (or the lack thereof) between doctors and patients was to use a wide-angle lens, as it were, to capture the broad picture. That "lens" was a brief questionnaire sent or administered to 3,000 physicians and patients across the country. The cohort included nephrologists and their patients (most of whom were on dialysis) as well as a broad range of physicians from diverse specialties and their patients, whose diagnoses were equally diverse. The sampling of both physicians and patients reflected a substantial minority (40 percent) of renal patients and nephrologists.

The brevity of the questionnaires and their anonymity (no identifying information or signatures were requested) were intended to encourage the recipients to complete them and to speak candidly. An overwhelming majority did so. Of the 2,743 forms that presumably reached their destination, more than 85 percent (2,392) were completed. (Two hundred seventy-four forms were returned for lack of a forwarding address or because the addressee was deceased.) Reflecting the high level of interest in the subject, some 20 percent of the respondents, chiefly physicians, added notes or letters to expand upon their responses.

Many of the surveys were administered individually by the author or by social workers in medical and dialysis clinics. The number of interviewers was limited to minimize the variability of interview skills. Responses were sorted by mail, self-administered, and administered surveys; however, since no significant differences emerged among the three types, aggregate data are reported here.

Patients were asked whether (1) they follow their doctor's instructions, (2) the doctor listens to their health concerns, (3) the doctor is usually available when needed, (4) they have enough time with the doctor to discuss their medical problems, and (5) how long they have to wait to see the doctor.

Physicians were asked whether (1) they believe patients follow instructions, (2) they listen to patients when they object to instructions, (3) they have modified treatment plans based on patient input, and (4) they feel constrained by regulatory influences such as insurers and health care regulators.

Both groups of respondents were invited to expand upon their answers and to complete the sentences "I wish my doctor (or patients) would..." and "I wish my doctor (or patients) would *not*...These wish lists are reproduced in

Table 2a

Survey

Patient Respondents	Total	Multi-Diagnosis (N=857)		Renal (N=572)	
		Urban	Rural	Urban	Rural
Number of respondents	1429	514	343	340	232
Age range	13-93	13-87	37-85	26-93	37-87
Average age	66	65	71	67	69
Male	629	231	133	159	106
Female	800	283	210	181	126
Non-white	487	170	04	185	28
With same MD for 5+ years	917	370	163	217	167

Responses:

	Total	Urban	Rural	Urban	Rural
Always follow instructions	657	63	174	244	176
Usually follow instructions	506	201	252	30	23
Do not follow instructions	327	194	84	40	9
Doctor listens	814	274	185	168	187
Doctor does not listen	491	182	126	156	27
Doctor is usually available	998	431	270	187	110
Doctor is not usually available	301	56	13	127	105
Ample time with doctor	946	365	291	209	81
Not enough time with doctor	340	82	27	120	111
Wait to see doctor: 1 day	614	262	161	122	69
Wait to see doctor: 1 week	482	200	82	108	92
Wait to see doctor: over 1 week	231	51	99	47	34

Table 2b

Survey

Physician Respondents	Total	Multi-Discipline (N=553)			Renal (N=370)	
		Urban	Suburban	Rural	Urban	Rural
Number of respondents	963	417	40	136	284	86
Male	711	290	37	118	204	62
Female	252	127	3	18	80	24
Non-white	341	100	0	66	103	72
In practice 5 years or less	318	147	4	25	128	14
In practice 6-15 years	406	231	26	19	112	18
In practice 16-25 years	217	83	7	26	75	23
In practice 25+ years	22	9	3	2	8	0
Care for 50 patients or less	113	49	0	23	26	15
Care for 51-99 patients	258	85	17	45	73	38
Care for 100-300 patients	307	141	23	23	100	20
Care for 301 or more patients	229	144	0	0	85	0
Responses:						
Patients follow instructions	354	187	8	64	66	29
Patients usually follow instructions	375	124	24	35	149	43
Patients never follow instructions	72	0	8	0	60	4
Doctor listens to patient objections	859	390	33	130	220	86
Doctor doesn't listen to patients	6	6	0	0	0	0
Doctor modifies treatment plans	770	284	33	117	249	87
Feels constrained by regulations	854	385	40	74	281	74
Setting:						
Free standing clinic	162	162	0	0	0	0
Hospital-based clinic	264	264	0	0	0	0
Private office	227	124	40	63	0	0
Chain-owned dialysis clinic	260	0	0	0	229	31
Private dialysis clinic	33	0	0	0	29	4
Government – owned dialysis clinic	6	0	0	0	6	0

Chapter 9, "In Their Own Words." Data regarding age, gender, race, and care setting were also collected. Tables 2a and 2b summarize the responses and the demography of the survey respondents.

Response to Questions

The greatest differential in responses occurred in the matter of physicians listening to patient complaints and patients following their doctors' instructions.

Nearly all the physicians (90 percent) reported that they "always listen" to patient complaints and 80 percent said they modify treatment plans accordingly. Only six physicians confessed that they don't listen to patients. Little more than half (57 percent) of the patients, on the other hand, believed their doctors listen to their concerns, and more than a third (nearly 500 in all or 34 percent) asserted that their doctors "do not listen." In the matter of following instructions, the tables were turned. Little more than one-third (38 percent) of the doctors (and only one-fourth of the nephrologists) felt their patients always followed instructions while nearly half the patients (and three-fourths of the renal patients) were convinced that they always complied with their doctor's instructions. The majority of both patients and doctors, however, agreed that most patients complied "always or most of the time."

Fewer than half (43 percent) of the patients are seen by their doctors within one day, but most (77 percent) are seen within one week after calling for an appointment. About one out of five patients, however, waits longer than a week to see a physician. Only about half (51 percent) of the renal patients, compared with three-fourths (77 percent) of those with multiple diagnoses considered that they have ample time with their physicians. One-fourth of all patients (and nearly half of the renal patients) stated that they did not have ample time with doctor to discuss their concerns.

Physicians were not asked directly about time spent with patients. They were, however, asked whether they felt "constrained by health care regulations." Their response was a resounding "Yes!" Overall, nine out of ten physicians felt constrained by the regulations, with only the multi-discipline practitioners in rural areas less adamant. (Only about half felt such constraints.) Many noted that costly co-payments, lack of prescription drug coverage or limited formularies, complicated referral systems, and repeated trips to hospital outpatient departments to satisfy reimbursement requirements contribute to patient non-compliance. Others acknowledged that they spend less time with patients because of the extensive paperwork required; furthermore, they reported, some managed care companies dictate the maximum amount of time to be spent with a patient. "HMOs direct patient care," one physician wrote, "no matter what anyone says."

Physicians felt that they are forced to practice "defensive and documentary" medicine to satisfy the insurers rather than the needs of the patients and that restrictive treatment guidelines causes them to become "creative" in filling out forms. Many respondents resented the "second-guessing" by insurance companies that limits prescription options to a restricted formulary. "I have to compromise my standards of care to meet insurance requirements," one physician commented.

In general, physicians saw communication with government regulators and managed care organizations as a key part of their communication problem with patients and called for a dialogue between physicians and regulators to address such issues as duplicative paperwork, denials of needed services, and inflexible rules that ignore the individual needs of patients.

Sample Demographics

Patients

Of the 1,429 patient respondents, 40 percent were dialysis patients. Nearly two-thirds (64 percent) had been with the same doctor for five years or more.

With an average age of 66, most patient respondents were experienced observers of the health care scene, but the ages ranged from 13 to 93. Slightly more than half (56 percent) were female, and one in three (34 percent) was African American, Asian, Indian, or Hispanic (reported as "non-white"). Among the renal patients, more than half of those in urban settings were non-white, compared to only 28 patients (12 percent) in rural areas.

Physicians

Of the total number of physician respondents (963), three-fourths practiced in urban areas and about one-fourth in rural communities. Suburban practices accounted for less than four percent. Nearly two-thirds (62 percent) were multi-specialty providers; slightly more than one-third (38 percent), renal specialists. The majority of physicians in all categories had been in practice for 15 years or less; however, about one in four reported practicing medicine for 16 years or longer.

In general, urban practitioners from all specialties tended to serve larger caseloads than their rural counterparts. (Half served 100 patients or more). The vast majority of nephrologists saw patients in chain-owned dialysis clinics, while most multi-specialty physicians were affiliated with hospital-based clinics or saw patients in a private office or freestanding clinic. All suburban respondents practiced in a private office.

Not surprisingly, the physician population was more male dominated (73 percent) and slightly more non-white (37 percent) than the patient group. Rural nephrologists represented the largest non-white proportion (84 percent).

Conclusion

In examining the responses, it may be tempting to view the "cup" as "half full." The majority of patients believe that their doctors listen to them, are usually available to them, and spend ample time with them, and the majority of physicians are confident that their patients follow instructions most of the time and are willing to modify treatment plans on the basis of patient input. That more than half the patients and physicians are relatively satisfied with their level of communication *is* positive. These individuals should be grateful for the quality of their interrelationships, and their colleagues and/or fellow patients can learn from their examples.

Equally important—indeed, perhaps more important—is the sizeable minority whose level of communication is less than optimal. A significant "disconnect" exists when, for example, 90 percent of physicians but only 57 percent of patients believe that doctors "always listen" to patient complaints. Particularly disconcerting is the 34 percent of patients—more than 500—who said flatly that their doctors *don't* listen to them and the 23 percent of all patients (and half of the renal patients) who feel that they do not have ample time to discuss their concerns with their physicians. Awareness of the "half-empty cup" is what prompted the writing of this book. These are the individuals who will benefit most from its contents, and their numbers are sufficiently large to justify a proactive approach to improving doctor-patient communications.

Particularly telling was the virtually unanimous consensus among physicians regarding the constraints imposed by health care regulators and managed care organizations. Their conviction that excessive restrictions are negatively impacting both the quality of care and the quality of doctor-patient relationships indicates the urgent need, articulated by several physicians, for a constructive dialogue with regulators about the most pressing problems.

The nearly 2400 patients and physicians who responded to the questionnaire confirmed that doctor-patient communication is an area that deserves a closer look—a more precise diagnosis and, perhaps, a course of treatment. That closer look came in the form of focus groups across the country and nearly 100 individual interviews. The next three chapters report findings from these investigations.

*My doctor always takes time to listen to me, and sometimes he
even agrees with me. I wish he would agree more often.*

(Patient)

*I am an individual. The doctor needs to recognize me as such. I
know my body better than he does.*

(Patient)

Response to the invitation to patients to participate in a
series of focus groups was most encouraging. In all, 375
patients took part in 35 group discussions in urban, rural,
and suburban settings in nine states: Pennsylvania, Ohio,
West Virginia, New Jersey, Georgia, Florida, California,
Illinois, and Michigan. One-third of the groups and nearly
half the participants were dialysis or transplant patients;
the remainder were from primary care, internal medicine,
oncology, cardiology, and endocrinology, and a few were
older pediatric patients who attended with their parents.

Focus group patient participants were significantly
more likely to see communication with their physicians as
a problem than were the physicians in focus groups or
physicians and patients who completed the survey. More
than two-thirds (68 percent) of the renal patients and more
than half (51 percent) of those from other diagnosis groups
said they did not communicate well with their physicians,

and about half of both groups believed that their physicians do not adequately listen to or address their concerns. More than half from each group faulted physicians for frequently changing prescriptions and thus placing a financial hardship on the patient. The area of greatest agreement with the physician focus groups concerned the negative impact of government and insurance company regulations on the quality of care they receive. Eighty percent of the renal patients and 70 percent of those with other diagnoses (compared with 97 percent of physician focus group participants) cited government and insurance regulations as a major concern and barrier to effective care. [See *Table 3*.]

Table 3. Demographics and Chief Concerns of Patient Focus Groups

Patient Focus Groups	Total	Multi-Diagnosis	Renal
Number of focus groups	35	23	12
Number of participants	375	224	151
Setting for group			
Urban	68%	63%	75%
Rural	23%	25%	20%
Suburban	9%	12%	5%
Average length of group discussion	90 minutes	90 minutes	90 minutes
Beliefs:			
Communication with doctor is poor	58%	51%	68%
Doctor doesn't listen	50%	47%	54%
Prescriptions are changed too often	60%	59%	62%
Regulations limit care	74%	70%	80%

Patients participated actively in the discussions, and in five cases, the session extended to two hours. In general, the rural groups were less vocal that those from urban areas. These participants were older, more hesitant to criticize their relationship with their physicians, and despite concern about treatments that they did not understand, their common response was "I guess the doctor knows best." Urban patients seemed more empowered to address issues without thought of repercussion. They were more outspoken, more critical, and less accepting of the demands of a busy medical practice. Of all the participants, however, renal patients were most critical of the doctor-patient relationships and faulted their nephrologists for lack of time, unclear explanations, and unwillingness to acknowledge or understand why the patients were sometimes noncompliant.

The majority of the patients acknowledged their physicians' competence while identifying specific concerns that, they felt, were undermining communication and interaction.

Time with the Patient

The physician's lack of time to discuss the patient's concerns and treatment was considered a primary concern by many patients. Patients described an "assembly line mentality" in physicians who scheduled patients at such short intervals that they had time only to "see the symptoms but not the patient." Many patients commented on physicians who have "too much paperwork," but on further questioning, it appeared that "paperwork" was the doctor's excuse for long waiting times or shortened visits. Some see the "assembly line" environment in clinics, dialysis units, and private offices as a way of increasing the physician's income. "They are making money so they don't care how long we wait," one patient observed. For some, however, time is not a problem. "My doctor always takes time to listen to me, and sometimes he even agrees with me," a patient reported, adding "I wish he would agree more often."

Courtesy

Many patients were offended by the lack of courtesy displayed by the physicians and their staffs, and some went so far as to call them "rude." They saw the long waiting times as discourteous and a signal that patients are not important and their time has no value. Some patients expressed the belief that the quality of their care was directly related to their income and their insurance coverage, and others said they were reluctant to complain or question their physician because they did not have private insurance, adding with a shrug, "You get what you pay for."

Patients interpreted the physician's "superior attitude" as still another indication of their own low station in life. Many cited the patronizing attitudes of both physicians and staff as the reason for their reluctance to seek clarification of information or instructions they did not understand. Some patients said their doctor "talked down" to them as if they were "stupid." "My doctor gives vague answers to my questions and then gets mad when I push for clearer answers," a patient said. "I'm not stupid; I just don't understand." Many patients remarked on the physician's irritation if they asked the same question more than once and suggested that some physicians view questions as an attack on their competence or a challenge to it. "Sometimes you have to read the doctor's mood before you ask questions," a patient observed. Another said, "My doctor works on a need-to-know basis. If he doesn't think you need to know or would not understand, then information is withheld."

Patients differed on the role of the doctor's staff members. "I wish my doctor would spend more time talking to me rather than sending messages to me by the nurse," one patient commented. Another had no objection to talking with the support staff. "I trust the nurses sometimes more than the doctor, " she said. "They know me and my case better than the doctor does." Several suggested that physicians in group practices sometimes fail to share information with their partners who may also care for a specific patient. "My doctor should discuss my case with his partners," a patient said. "They don't have a clue about my care. When they fill in for him, they ask questions that are answered in my chart."

Sensitivity to Patients' Needs

Patients stated that their physician was not sensitive to the issues that caused them to be noncompliant—for example, lack of funds for transportation to the clinic or inadequate insurance coverage for prescriptions. Some patients said their doctors "don't have a clue" about the patient's income and often prescribe medications without regard to their insurance coverage. Patients suggested that samples be used more often to determine the patient's tolerance for new medications before prescribing them. "My doctor should consider and discuss side effects of medication before I buy medicine that I can't take," one patient remarked.

Privacy and confidentiality were issues with many patients. Physicians were criticized for asking personal questions in the clinic setting and repeating the answers in a loud voice that could be overheard by other patients. Physicians' staff members, patients reported, often repeated patient information in areas where others could overhear it.

Several patients observed that physicians seem to have forgotten the importance of drawn curtains in exam areas.

Younger patients were concerned about physician office hours. They complained that the physicians' office hours often make it difficult for them to attend to their health needs without jeopardizing their employment. Many stated they delayed seeking care until symptoms worsened because office hours were inconvenient.

Dialysis patients discussed at great length the "difficult patient" and the unwillingness of many nephrologists to address behaviors that impacted on the quality of other patients' lives during treatment. They believed that the doctors' failure to intervene was, in a sense, giving the "difficult" patient permission to continue that behavior and to cause an already unpleasant environment to become even more so. Dialysis patients also felt that nephrologists often unfairly attributed the need for access revisions to patient noncompliance when, in fact, the problem was the physician's competence rather than the patient's compliance.

Some multi-diagnosis patients were more cavalier about compliance. "I follow my doctor's instructions if they make sense," one patient explained. "If they don't, I change my dose according to how I feel. I know my body better than the doctor does." Others resented the physician's habit of comparing one patient to another. "I am an individual," one remarked. "He needs to recognize me as such." Another patient expressed her resentment at being told, "You're not as sick as you think you are." She added, "My doctor is painfully honest. He is almost cruel in his honesty. He says 'Do it or die. It's up to you.' He could use some lessons in tact."

Doctor/Patient Partnerships

Patient complaints and criticisms can be extremely informative to health care providers who are truly committed to improving their communication and relationship with their patients. Equally informative, however, are the statements of praise, of love, and of loyalty that came from many of the focus group participants. Even those who had a specific complaint often qualified it with an expression of respect, confidence, or affection for the physician. If the criticisms can be used as "don'ts," these spontaneous comments can serve equally well as a "do" list for doctors, their office staff, and health providers throughout the system.

Good relationships don't happen over night. As one patient said, "It takes time to find a comfort level with a new doctor. Until I can really trust my doctor, I can't tell him half the things he needs to know to make an accurate diagnosis."

Sometimes relationships are built on sharing personal information. "I see pictures of my doctor's family, especially the prom and wedding pictures and new grandchildren," a patient said. "They make me feel like a member of the family." Another added, "My doctor does a lot for me. He really cares about me and my family."

Other patient observations included:

"My doctor doesn't know how much I love him. He keeps me alive."

"My doctor looks into my soul and helps me make it through the day."

"My doctor treats me with great respect; I love him for it."

"My doctor is a savior."

"My doctor is responsive to me, not reactionary."

"My doctor and me have a give-and-take relationship: he respects me and I respect him."

"My doctor and I are a team. We take good care of me."

"Listen to the patient," Sir William Osler told his medical students a century ago. "He's telling you what's wrong with him." To that good advice, I would add: "Listen to the patient: he's telling you what's wrong (and what's right) about your relationship. He's telling you how to communicate with him."

Physician Focus Groups
From the Other End of the Stethoscope

4

I love it when my patients listen to my questions and respond with honest answers. I love patients who love themselves enough to take care of themselves.

(Doctor)

I wish patients would not demand treatment based on what their neighbors, friends, TV, or their mothers tell them and judge the appropriateness of my advice on the basis of what others say.

(Doctor)

Physicians greeted the invitation to participate in a series of focus groups with great interest. In all, 187 physicians attended 25 group sessions in urban and rural areas of Pennsylvania, Georgia, Ohio, Florida, New York, Maryland, California, Illinois, and Washington, DC. Nine of the focus groups (45 percent) included nephrologists only; the remaining 16 (55 percent) included practitioners from various disciplines including primary care, endocrinology, emergency medicine, surgery, pediatrics, and obstetrics/gynecology. The groups ranged from five to nine members and lasted for 45 minutes to two hours. Average time was 90 minutes.

In contrast to the participants in the patient focus groups, less than half of whom felt they communicated well with their physicians, nearly three-fourths (72 percent) of the physicians said they believed they communicated well with most patients. Almost as many (70 vs. 72 percent) also believed that their patients communicate well whereas half the patient participants said their doctors "don't listen." While about three-fourths (74 percent) of patients felt that regulations imposed by the government and insurance carriers limited access to "good care," nearly all the physicians (97 percent) agreed that these regulations placed unreasonable restraints on their delivery of health care.

Table 4. Demographics and Chief Concerns of Physician Focus Groups

Physician Focus Groups	Total
Number of focus groups	25
Number of participants	187
Setting for group	
Urban	71%
Rural	19%
Suburban	10%
Average length of group discussion	90 minutes
Beliefs:	
Communicate well with most patients	72%
Patients communicate well with MD	70%
Medical decisions made by non-MDs	62%
Regulations limit care	97%

In all the groups, physicians were candid and willing to share very personal issues and concerns. Their caring and concern for the well being of their patients was evident, and many of the comments reiterated statements made on the written surveys. The focus groups afforded the physicians an opportunity to expand upon their concerns. Several consistent themes related to communication emerged across all groups.

Impact of Regulations

Physicians noted that regulatory agencies and insurance companies often impact negatively on their ability to deliver good health care. Regulations, they believed, restricted their options in delivering care they considered necessary, and a significant number (62 percent) commented on their frustration when medical decisions were dictated by non-physicians or physicians who no longer practiced in the clinical arena. Some physicians suggested that patients should become more political to advocate on their own behalf with insurance companies and government agencies for more adequate funding and legislation that afforded physicians opportunities to practice medicine in the way that they were trained.

Physicians also believed that the inordinate amount of "paper work" required by governmental agencies and insurance carriers took time away from the business of caring for patients. Some, however, expressed surprise that patients do not believe they were given enough time to discuss their medical problems or concerns. They consider the time they must devote to "endless" paperwork as an extension of care for their patients. Those who acknowledged that lack of time sometimes contributes to barriers of communication admitted that their behavior may have made it appear that they were too busy or preoccupied to listen to the patient. When they were aware of a problem, they said, they sought follow-up conversation to establish the needed communication link.

Patient Attitudes and Behaviors

Some physicians expressed with surprising candor their frustration and anger at their patients' inability to understand the severity of their illness and the importance of following prescribed treatments. Several commented on the unwillingness of patients to take responsibility for their own health. Patients who listen (that is, comply with instructions and ask more questions when they were not clear on information provided by the doctor), experience better outcomes, the physicians believe. Some stressed that patients should recognize the importance of keeping scheduled appointments and reschedule if they are unable to keep appointments. The physicians believe that many patients fail to understand that their health status is dependent upon regular physician interaction.

Other Communication Issues

Most physicians welcomed patients' efforts to learn more about their illness but cautioned that it is important for patients to discuss their newfound information with their physicians to assure clear understanding. They also cautioned that patients should not depend upon the Internet for second opinions or make decisions based on Internet information without benefit of consultation with their physicians. Similarly, they pointed out, patients should not assume that the advice they overhear given to another patient is necessarily applicable to their particular illness.

Many physicians agreed that they miss much of the nonverbal body language that signals a problem with the patients. They cited a patient "blow-up" as often the first clue to communication problems. One physician described his follow-up calls placed at dinnertime to evidence his concern. These calls, he believed, say in action as well as in words that the patient is important.

Expectations and Assumptions

Discussion of patient expectations and assumptions was quite lively in all the groups. When told that many patients had criticized the care given by a group practice physician's partners in the absence of their own doctor, the immediate response was to dismiss these concerns as unfounded. Physicians reacted positively, however, when an orientation to the practice was suggested for all patients, new and current. They acknowledged that patients need to understand how the group practice works and that they should be assured that standards of care would be adhered to, no matter which physician was seen.

Unreasonable expectation of cure posed a problem for many of the physicians. One said candidly that doctors often feel inadequate in their inability to cure the patient but fail to admit their fears or their inadequacies. Many physicians expressed concern that far too many patients were adept at transferring ownership and responsibility for illness to the physician with an expectation of resolution, and they found themselves becoming apologists for the disease while the patients "sat back and waited for the cure." Most participants agreed that many patients have unrealistic images of the "supernatural ability to cure." One physician said it best: "I am not Marcus Welby. Marcus Welby is dead. I cannot hear the complaint and cure the disease in fifty minutes."

Doctor/Patient Partnerships

Most physicians supported the concept of a partnership with their patients, with each partner responsible for specific components of the treatment plan and accountable to the "partnership." They agreed that developing an open dialogue was essential to establishing a partnership. Others felt that the concept of a partnership was difficult for some patients and physicians to embrace. Much discussion centered on the "newness" of the idea that doctors expect patients to take an active role in the treatment regimen.

Some physicians discussed the necessity of taking the time to treat the whole person as well as the sick patient. Patients must understand that the real power of the partner relationship and its effectiveness is in their hands, some physicians believe.

One pediatrician discussed his approach to building rapport with his young patients. He said that he wore funny ties with a shirt, never scrubs, during an office visit so that he would look like a "regular" guy and patients would see him as a person, rather than just as a doctor, and discover "the child in me." He asks older patients if they wished to have their parents present during the exam, and he makes an effort to tell patients what they need to know in terms that they and their parents can understand. He tells patients when their actions make him angry and explains what it takes for them to work together. He also invites patients to tell him they are angry. He finds that open dialogue, with the terms of the relationship stated and mutually agreed upon goals, assures good communication.

Another pediatrician, who is chief of pediatric surgery, suggested that physicians would be advised to change the golden rule from "Do unto others, as you would have them do unto you" to the "platinum rule": "Do unto others as they would want done to them." As difficult as it sometimes is to accept, he pointed out, physicians must, after providing appropriate information, accept patients' informed decisions on how and when they will receive care.

The Interviews
Up Close and Personal

5

Physicians must remember that non-compliance is a patient's right.

(Doctor)

'Dr. Doorknob' is always on his way out the door. When he tries to calm me down, he's a day late and a dollar short.

(Patient)

They tried to take away my hope, and I said, "No way!" I am a miracle in progress.

(Doctor as Patient)

From both the surveys and the focus groups, it became apparent that physicians and patients had much to say about their communication with each other. It was also apparent that, in many cases, the succinct format of the questionnaire and the time-limited focus groups were leaving part of the story untold. Some appended notes or even letters to their questionnaires, but because the survey was anonymous, follow-up was impossible. Some focus group participants seemed hesitant to speak out in the presence of their peers, while other were still eager to share their experiences after two hours. Consequently, to flesh out the unfolding story, I undertook a third approach to information gathering: open-ended, private one-on-one interviews with physicians, other health care professionals, and patients. In all, 92 in-depth interviews were conducted, and a sampling of the responses (about 25 percent of the total) is reported here. They are reflective of the total complement and particularly expressive of the frustrations experienced by all three cohorts of respondents.

The interviews, which averaged 90 minutes, ranged from 30 minutes to three hours. They were conducted in private physician offices, ambulatory care settings, or in private homes. Regardless of the setting, the respondents welcomed the opportunity to discuss their health care experiences and, in the private setting, spoke with great candor and conviction. All recognized the general lack of effective communication and the urgent need to develop strategies for improving hearing and listening skills.

This chapter summarizes the representative interviews in three sections:

- **Health Care Professionals as Patients**—physicians and other providers who find themselves at the other end of the stethoscope. These individuals should have known how to provide and elicit the information needed to create an environment of enlightened communication. In many cases, however, the conflict between expectation and assumption left them with a sense of frustration and helplessness that is normally considered the lot of patients without medical training.

- **Health Care Professionals as Providers**—physicians and other providers who approach patients in widely divergent ways. Some displayed their frustrations and vulnerability in their view of questions as a form of confrontation and their conviction that patient non-compliance is a universal problem. Some cited the negative impact of non-verbal communication, while others saw good communication as a vital component of prevention. Several addressed obvious health disparities in the minority community, emphasizing the variation in cultural competencies (patients' and physicians') as well as economic and educational deficiencies. Some freely acknowledged the need for providers to become better listeners and more skilled at providing adequate and understandable information. One identified "I don't know" as a way for physicians to share with patients their "humanness" in health care.

- **Patients as Patients**—expressions of frustration and anger at failing to get the information and guidance they need from physicians as well as deep and abiding appreciation and love for those physicians who are teachers and those who share the pain with their patients.

Health Care Professionals as Patients

Subject: Female physician specializing in obstetrics
and gynecology
Race: Caucasian
Diagnosis: Benign brain tumor

*After several months of unexplained headaches, the patient was
referred to a neurologist and neurosurgeon by her primary care
physician. She was assured that the surgery should be uneventful
and that she could expect short-term disability of six to eight
weeks. She was informed of the slight risk of death but was assured
that it was a remote possibility. The surgeon did not mention the
risk of paralysis or stroke. In reality, three and half years after the
operation, this patient is not able to return to her practice. She has
a severe speech impediment; she has suffered several strokes and is
able to walk short distances only with assistance.*

Although the patient considers her morbidity to be a
consequence of the surgery, she has never discussed her
frustration with her surgeon because she is grateful that
her life was saved due to the surgery. "The benign tumor
pressed on my thalamus, and my heart could have
stopped," she explained. Despite her loss, she maintains an
upbeat outlook on life and believes in "grabbing life and
squeezing it everyday."

During the course of several hour-long interviews, the
patient shared her thoughts about her own experiences as

a patient and as a doctor and offered some suggestions for improving communications with patients.

"Physicians who cared for me expected me to know all about my condition and took short cuts in the discussions," she said. "They assumed that I would ask questions, but I did not know

> "I did not know enough to ask the right questions. The doctors had forgotten that I was out of my specialty."

enough to ask the right questions. The doctors had forgotten that I was out of my specialty." By contrast, she described her primary care physician as "loving and kind, an excellent communicator—he listens to me and I listen to him."

She believes that doctors need to "tell it like it is." They should tell the patient the truth, not paint a pretty picture. And, she believes, when the news is bad, they must understand that "the patient stops listening and it will be necessary to repeat the information more than once to make sure the patient heard and understood the information." When she was in practice, she recalled, "the more experience I gained, the more comfortable I became in saying, 'I don't know—but I will try to find out.'" She is convinced that "patients appreciate that kind of honesty and will trust your judgment. An informed patient is what I strived for in my practice…Physicians must remember that they were people before they became physicians."

Despite her diminished physical capacities, this patient looks to the future with great optimism. She believes she has the responsibility to help others, particularly as an advocate for women with disabilities. "I know that my brain works fine," she explains, "but society is prejudiced against people who do not speak well. Patients with disabilities must be given opportunity for access to good health care." She serves on an advisory board for a large women's hospital that has developed an ambulatory care program for disabled women and reviews articles for clinical suitability for the advisory board of a professional journal. She also plans to develop a web site to answer ob/gyn questions for women. For her continuing contributions to medicine, her local medical society recognized her as "Primary Care Physician of the Year" during her rehabilitation.

She admits that the adjustment has not been easy, for herself or for her family. *(See comments from her physician husband, page 40.)* "It was difficult to accept the fact that I would never deliver another baby. . . . They said I would not walk and I am walking. They said I would not talk and I am talking. They tried to take away my hope and I said, 'No way!'" But she is sustained by the hope that she can continue to use her medical knowledge in new areas. She will use her time to "broaden her horizons" through reading, travel, and writing about her experiences on her road to recovery. "I am a miracle in progress," she states with confidence.

The husband's view

Subject: **Male physician, a specialist in pulmonary medicine, and husband of the patient in the previous interview.**

This physician consented to an interview to reflect upon his experience as the husband of a physician spouse who underwent surgery with catastrophic outcomes. He spoke with great candor on how this experience had affected the entire family and how it had caused him to re-evaluate and rethink his relationship with his patients.

The physician said that neither he nor his wife had communicated their expectations relative to the surgery or its outcome. In retrospect, he believed that the surgeon had not been realistic in describing the possible outcomes—possibly on the assumption that the couple understood the risks because they were physicians. Consequently, when the surgeon's optimistic predictions proved to be inaccurate, the patient and her family were unprepared for the outcome, shocked, and angry. A once healthy, viable respected physician had become a patient with limited speech, unable to walk, and with some cognitive deficit. The neurological impairment necessitated a complete treatment plan—medical, psychiatric, and physical rehabilitation.

Their teenage daughters found it most difficult to accept their mother's illness and the changes in family life that it necessitated. The husband described his own need to "get

Physicians must give patients the information they need, he said, "in a straight forward way, without sugar-coating the bad news." The condescending attitude of some physicians, he added, "is a turn-off and causes patients to become non-communicative." So does over-familiarity, he said: "Don't call me 'honey'—call me by my name." He is pleased with what he sees at his hospital in terms of patient-doctor interaction: "Our doctors model appropriate communication skills for the doctors in training." One way to do this during hospital rounds, he pointed out, is to "make sure that the patient is the center of the discussion."

In his own relationships with physicians, both personal and professional, he has found that some doctors assumed, because of his health care background, that he knew more than he actually did. He has never hesitated, however, to ask for clarification. As a social worker, he sees his role as helping patients cope with their illness and learn to communicate with their physicians to become informed consumers. He stressed the importance of patient responsibility for embracing the care plan and being compliant. "What you know can help you," he said. "What you don't know can kill you."

> **"What you know can help you. What you don't know can kill you."**

Subject: Female nurse anesthetist (retired)

Race: African American

Diagnosis: Chronic arthritis and cancer

After suffering from debilitating arthritis that forced her into private practice to allow a more flexible schedule, this patient developed cancer ten years ago after minor breast reduction surgery. The lump she found at the incision site was initially misdiagnosed as an infection. A second opinion confirmed her suspicion of cancer. Three surgeries and chemotherapy followed the diagnosis. Complications from knee surgery resulted in a life-threatening episode of gangrene.

Like the previous patient, she described the dialogue with most of her physicians as colleague-to-colleague rather than as patient-to-physician and expressed the feeling

> **Angry at misdiagnosis? "No, God led me to the second surgeon."**

that, overall, she had had an excellent relationship with a series of physicians over the last 20 years. She, too, acknowledged the role of faith in her recovery. Asked whether she was angry with the first surgeon (who misdiagnosed her cancer), she replied, "No, God led me to the second surgeon." "God has his own way of showing you what is important," she believes, and she asked Him to allow her to keep her spirit so that she could manage her illness.

On prompting, she acknowledged great disappointment in the "careless" manner in which her complaints and symptoms were handled prior to the diagnosis of cancer, and she attributed the "misadventure" with her knee surgery to the surgeon "who was in a hurry."

In remission for a number of years, cancer recurred recently in a new site, and the patient is again in treatment.

Health Care Professionals as Providers

Subject: Male physician
Race: Caucasian
Specialty: Pulmonary medicine

(This is a continuation of the interview with the husband of the physician-patient who suffered catastrophic outcomes after surgery for a benign brain tumor. Here he speaks in more general terms about the barriers to communication faced by practicing physicians.)

The physician identified time and money as significant barriers to communication. Paperwork and documentation are time-consuming but essential to justify payment, he said, but they steal valuable time from doctor/patient conferences. "I detest the amount of time I must take to do paperwork for insurance companies," he said, "The allotted time with patients is insufficient, and we are forced to perform highly focused exams (addressing chiefly the patients' presenting complaints) due to time constraints."

Patients, on the other hand, don't always understand that physicians have time constraints, and he believes they must learn to focus on the doctor's questions and answer them

> **"Physicians must remember that non-compliance is a patient's right."**

completely but concisely. He emphasized the need to maximize the available time for meaningful dialogue between physician and patient. He acknowledged that patients expect "face time" with the physician—time to be seen and heard during the visit. He described his group practice as "unique" because it allots one half hour per patient visit, compared to the 15 minutes allotted by most HMOs. A university setting allows this luxury, he said.

Another potential barrier, he said, can be the patient's level of intelligence and knowledge. This must determine the physician's approach, and it is imperative for the physician to "keep things simple." Patients are aware when physicians make the effort to speak on the patient's level of understanding, he said. "Common sense dictates 'plain talk.'" This, however, does not mean "talking down" to patients. He detests the patronizing attitude of some physicians and believes that it can discourage patients from communicating their fears and concerns.

To ensure that patients understand and remember the information given by physicians, he suggested that patients take notes on the conversation. When patients are referred to new physicians, they should be advised by the referring physician to list all medications (prescription and non-prescription) for the new physician's information.

Pointing out that hearing and listening are different, he stressed that both patients and physicians should share their expectations to avoid misunderstanding and dissatisfaction. "I diffuse unrealistic expectations," he said, "even though that may involve telling patients things they don't want to hear." He believes that instructions to patients

should be succinct to encourage compliance, but he pointed out that physicians must remember that non-compliance is a patient's right."

Subject: **Female physician**
Race: **African American**
Specialty: **Internal Medicine**

*As chair of the Department of Family Medicine in a university
medical school, this physician spoke chiefly to the health disparities
identified in the minority community and the importance of communication in improving the quality of care.*

Addressing the importance of providing adequate
resources to ensure that patients who have been labeled as
socially downtrodden and disadvantaged achieve equity in
the receipt of health care services, she said it is imperative
to train clinicians who are prepared to provide care to all
segments of the population. She noted that her role as
teacher in the medical school offers numerous opportunities
to effect needed change. "I truly believe that one person can
be instrumental in causing positive change," she said. "I
would like to be seen as 'knightess for change.' Effective
communication is a learned behavior which must be
embraced by all."

Communication and listening skills must become inte-
grated into life experience, she believes. "Communication
problems are a direct result of individuals looking at a sit-

uation through a different lens, colored by differences in cultural, racial, or economic background. Most physicians, she said, listen from their own personal experiences and perspective, which are

> **"Non-compliance is a failure of the system in non-recognition of the psycho-social impediments."**

often very different from those of the patients they treat. When patients do not keep appointments and are labeled as failed or non-compliant patients, physicians must recognize this as a failure of our system in the non-recognition of the psychosocial impediments, which often preclude compliance. She shared many instances where poor communication between physicians and patients was identified and appropriate strategies were developed to provide positive outcomes.

The physician has a responsibility to help patients understand how the health care system is structured so that they can successfully access the system. Using the analogy of the "Gardener's Tale" to describe disparities in the delivery of health care, she said, "A seed that is watered and nurtured will blossom into a flower; a seed without the same care will not blossom. Similarly, patients who do not receive equal care and treatment will have negative outcomes. The environment in which care is provided is very critical to positive outcomes."

Subject: Male dental surgeon
Race: Arabian
Specialty: Prosthodontics

This health care provider specializes in crowns, bridges, dentures, implant, and reconstructive dentistry.

Identifying "good communication" as the cornerstone of effective treatment, this surgeon stressed the importance of forming a partnership with his patients in which each partner is

> **"Good communication is the cornerstone of effective treatment."**

"clear" on his or her responsibilities. He described his practice: "I *listen* to the patient describe symptoms and concerns, then I *educate* the patient on the probable cause of symptoms and allay concerns related to the actual treatment process; then I *treat* the patient."

He was convinced that the need for preventive care has not been stressed enough in minority communities since a disproportionate portion of his patients presented with avoidable dental problems. He discussed the need for closer collaboration between the dental and medical resources in the community, noting that the dental community had "dropped the ball" in terms of placing the necessary emphasis on preventive care.

"A child who is taught to care for teeth and gums seldom finds his way into my office as an adult," he said.

Subject: Male physician/chief medical officer
Race: Caucasian
Specialty: Internal Medicine

This tenured medical school professor is on staff of a large university-affiliated teaching hospital. The demographics of the hospital's service area includes a large geriatric area.

This physician believes patients should be encouraged to learn about their illness through a variety of resources (i.e., pamphlets, books, the Internet) and to validate what they

> "A test of wills between doctor and patient causes a delay in diagnosis and treatment."

learn with their physicians in order to move toward "owning" responsibility for their care. Although some patients do not have the capacity or ability to do so, those who are able to own the disease are more likely to be compliant.

He says that physicians need to "get into the head of the patients" to determine how the patients' daily experience will impact on their ability to be compliant. Patients must be encouraged to self manage their care. The physician must be able to communicate clearly in language they understand. Patients must be taught to understand that they have the ultimate responsibility for the management of their illness.

Geriatric patients are good candidates for self-management, he believes. Once they own the disease, they are taught to manage and make the necessary life-style accommodations, and they are able to self-manage much better. He discussed the development of a paradigm for geriatric population: How can we pay for the geriatrician to spend more "teaching time," which will result in less hospitalization? He described the ultimate patient care team—physician, health education nurse, pharmacist, dietician, and exercise therapist. The problem: There is no money to support such care.

"You have to reach patients where they are in terms of their understanding," he said. "The physician must make this determination as quickly as possible to begin the reciprocal education experience."

The physician discussed the need to personalize care for patients, addressing the individual needs of the patient. Patients need to share their personal home situations so that physician will be able to determine the probability of patient compliance. A test of wills between doctor and patient causes a delay in diagnosis and treatment.

In terms of the psychosocial interaction between physician and patient, he said that if he could dictate medical school admission criteria, he would insist that medical school candidates have real world experience. To gain patient trust must be a priority at the onset of a patient doctor relationship. The doctor's body language must communicate that the doctor is ready, willing, and able to provide care. The human connection must become a bridge to communicate.

Acquiring socio-economic information is essential to understanding "who" the patient is, he said. Cultural differences in house staff as they relate to a diverse patient population are critical to patient interaction. Urban teaching hospitals must take responsibility to provide pertinent information with reference to the many social systems that present for care. The defensiveness of some foreign national physicians "shuts off" communication with patients, he said, although female foreign national physicians appear to bridge the cultural gap with patients with more ease than their male counterparts.

All physicians must become more comfortable with the acknowledgement of "I don't know" as a matter of course. The doctor needs to say to the patient, "Usually such symptoms suggest _____ as a diagnosis, but I will check a number of areas by clinical test before I can make a final diagnosis." The patient will accept a delay in a final diagnosis if the doctor takes the time to explain the procedures."

Subject: **Male physician**
Race: **African American**
Specialty: **Internal medicine, gerontology, dentistry**

This physician, well past normal retirement age, is reluctant to give up his practice because of limited physician coverage in the community he serves. On the staff of an urban community health initiative of a major university health system, he sees many geriatric patients.

The physician discussed the need for clear and concise instructions to patients, saying that he often asks patients to repeat his instructions to be sure they understand what he has told them. When feasible, he encourages patients to have family members accompany them to the office visit.

Bemoaning the shortage of young physicians who are interested in gerontology, he reported some of his observations from his own practice. Older patients, he found, tend to over-medicate themselves because they become confused about the directions. He said that he also watches for signs of depression, which is common in older patients, in order to alert family members.

He believes in seeing the patient as a person rather than as "a coronary case" or "a hernia." In his practice, office visits are social affairs for the patients, and he deliberately schedules older patients on days when they are likely to see friends and can "visit" in the waiting room.

"My older patients love life," he said. "They accept the physical limitations caused by the aging process, and they look forward to tomorrow with hope."

> "My older patients love life....They look forward to tomorrow with hope."

Subject: Male physician
Race: Caucasian
Specialty: Nephrology

This nephrologist practices in a physician group which provides care to a large urban population. The patients are seen in a hospital-based dialysis clinic.

As a nephrologist, the physician is concerned about patient non-compliance. "Patients seem not to understand that end-stage renal disease has only two viable options—dialysis or transplantation," he said. "The third option is death, and that is due to non-compliance."

> **"ESRD has only two viable options—dialysis or transplantation. The third option is death."**

His expectations of his patients are clear: "Motivated patients who want to learn must understand they must be patient in the learning process. Patients are expected to be willing to ask questions and listen for the answer." To assure that his patients understand the information provided, he asks them to repeat the information he gives them. Patients are encouraged to bring written questions to meetings with the physician.

The establishment of good working relationships with patients is time-consuming and often emotionally draining, he admitted. "Patient non-compliance is a touchy topic, and I just don't have the time to fight with the patient."

Subject: Male physician/Director of a group practice
Race: Caucasian
Specialty: Internal Medicine

This internist practices in a large urban university-affiliated hospital. His group consists of five physicians, including two female practitioners. The patient population is middle class and white.

The physician focused on the obstacles to care that are created by patients by asking friends and relatives to validate treatment plans prescribed by the physician. Based on information gathered from those sources, he said, some patients stop or modify treatments or medications without consulting with their doctors.

Other patients, he believes, impede final diagnosis by presenting with too many symptoms and are not able to prioritize or define the severity of the symptoms. It is very difficult for patients to focus and prioritize. The physician must take a leadership role in directing the patient's attention to key issues.

Patients' complaints of physician lack of attention are valid, he feels. "Patients are often interrupted after twenty seconds of symptom description. I try really hard to keep quiet long enough for the patient to describe his symptoms."

The physician discussed the importance of family, friends, or significant others who are involved in the care plans. Involved family members facilitate the necessary compliance to a proposed treatment plan.

Noting that patients often comment on the rude treatment they receive from the office staff, he acknowledged that negative staff interaction with patients is a source of physician concern. In-service

> "I try really hard to keep quiet long enough for the patient to describe his symptoms."

programs have been initiated to improve patient satisfaction. Medical assistants are intended to assist in effective communication with patients but never to replace physician contact. He believes that patients must be afforded ample opportunities to discuss their concerns and to ask questions. Patients should not feel they must rush to share information.

The physician discussed the unique requirements to be observed when physicians provide care for other physicians. The temptation to socialize during the office visit must be minimized to focus on the reason for the visit. Physicians should err on the side of providing too much information rather than too little information.

Subject: Male physician
Race: Caucasian
Specialty: Nephrology

This physician is in a group that includes nephrologists, endocrinologists, and primary care physicians. The patient population includes urban/suburban individuals and families.

This physician envisions the doctor/patient relationship as an on-going play:

- Each person enters the scene with a prescribed role.

- Each player's unique background (age, sex, ethnicity, intellectual and emotional characteristics) is brought into play in the interaction between players. The patient's experience with the medical care system will impact on this relationship.

Patient might display anger, which has nothing to do with the doctor. The doctor must be able to read the cues and search for reasons for the displayed behavior.

> **In the drama of health care, doctors and patients play their own unique roles.**

He might be hurried due to an emergency and project annoyance that was not caused by the patient. All of these factors will influence the interactions.

Physicians must be alert to the body language and non-verbal communication which often tell more than verbal communication: non-response to introduction by physician, eye-avoidance, personal grooming, posture, odor, body movements, and yes/no answers.

The physician follows his script: history and physical examination. He must be directive in conversation with patient and prepared to give results of the examination to the patient as soon as possible. The physician must respond in words that the patient will understand.

In keeping with the play analogy, the play ends with dual climax: the physician climax is the provision of a diagnosis; the patient climax is the receipt of the diagnosis.

Patient peace of mind is the responsibility of the physician. Patients need to be reassured that the physician will do all in his power to make a definitive diagnosis. As one patient observed, "I care if the news is bad. I care even more when I don't know."

Subject: **Male physician**
Race: **African American**
Specialty: **Pediatric surgery**

The physician is on the staff of a major urban teaching hospital, which admits children from neonatal to age 18.

The physician is committed to establishing a trusting relationship with both child and parent because this will encourage parent and child to support each other in the relationship with physician. When possible, he wears a business suit rather than scrubs for his first meeting with the child. At this time, he also focuses on expectations—his and those of the family.

"The patient and family must understand that the power of the relationship is in their hands," he said. When he senses that the communication is not clear or acceptable, he supplements the communi-

> "I am not Marcus Welby, M.D. . . . I am not able to meet, diagnose, and cure within 50 minutes."

nication with a follow-up telephone call. He encourages his patients to express their concerns, anger, and frustrations. He also enjoys the same privileges he extends, sharing in laymen's terms his concerns and frustration as not always being able to "cure" the problem.

He believes that he operates on the Platinum Rule: "Do unto others, as they would want done to them." His interpretation of the Rule dictates telling family members and/or patients information when they are prepared, emotionally and mentally, to receive it. He stressed the need to repeat information as often as necessary to assure a full understanding of the diagnosis and available treatment options. Patients and families are the major components in the treatment options, he said, and successful relationships demand active communication and participation.

"I am not Marcus Welby, M.D. (a former television medical series)," he said. "The patient and family must understand that I am not able to meet, diagnose, and cure within 50 minutes or during our first encounter."

Subject: **Male physician/county health department medical director**
Race: **Caucasian**
Specialty: **Internal medicine/public health**

This physician, medical director of a large urban public health department, has benefited from exposure to an economically and culturally diverse population of patients and is able to see the health care system from their point of view as well as from that of the practicing physician.

Acknowledging that "good communication is the determinant factor in relationships between doctor and patient," the physician, however, cautioned that "patients and doctors must earn trust from each other before good communication may begin. A patient must believe that the doctor cares about him as a human being before he is willing to 'buy in' to the proposed diagnosis and treatment regime. And the physician must commit to learning about the patient's life and environment so that treatment plan is realistic and 'in tune' with patient lifestyle." He stressed that family involvement (including the extended family) is a critical component of successful interaction with the family.

Teaching, he believes, is an important part of the physician's role. "It is critical to encourage patients to learn as much as possible about their illness so that they can become active partners in the treatment," he said. "But it is also important to base expectations for participation on the patients' intellectual and emotional ability to do so."

Physicians must learn not to see questions as challenges and not view such dialogues as confrontation, he advised. "The three hardest words for a physician to say are 'I don't know,'" he said. "The failure to make this admission often serves as the beginning of mistrust by the patient, who does not understand the delay in diagnosis. Many patients, particularly minorities and the economically disadvantaged, fail to understand the benefits of continuity of care, and a trusted physician can help them to do so."

Non-compliance can be positive, he said. "Sometimes when a patient does not listen to my advice, that turns out to be a wise decision, particularly when the patient has withheld information that would have changed the advice given. Health care encompasses the whole patient—body and soul. Respect must be reciprocal: you must give respect to receive it. Class, title, and status are not the criteria for respect; it must be earned."

He warned that relationships between referring physicians and consultants are in need of much clearer definition. "Often the consultants share information with patients without a follow-up conversation with the referring physician," he said. "The result places patients in the middle of the physicians' 'battling egos.'"

Finally, he said, "Physicians must take the time to review their prescribing practices and use time as an ally. Often doctors prescribe medications too quickly. Doctors should view and treat patients in

> **"Sometimes when a patient does not listen to my advice, that turns out to be a wise decision."**

three general categories: acutely ill: reduce the severity; chronically ill: don't rush to prescribe until you determine that the patient can afford prescription changes; and life threatening: act quickly and hospitalize immediately.

Subject: Male physician
Race: Caucasian
Specialty: Nephrology

This physician practiced medicine, specializing in nephrology, for more than 30 years before his death shortly after this interview was conducted.

A veteran of both a university health care setting and a government-operated hospital system, he observed that the two systems were more similar than dissimilar. He cited the great amount of paper work and the over-scheduling of patients as deterrents to good patient care. "The patients get caught in the middle," he said. "I sometimes think that both sides forget about the patient."

The physician stated that he went into medicine to help patients but found the growing bureaucracy a great problem that needs to be addressed. His treatment philosophy is based on giving each patient as much time as is needed. Some, he said, want to know as little as possible; others want to know everything. "You have to take the time to know your patient, mind and body, to provide the best possible care," he said.

What does he expect from his patients? "Honesty," he replied, explaining that he encourages patients to talk with him and not to withhold information. "It's a long process," he said, "and I have to model the behavior I expect from the patients."

> "If patients and doctors don't commit to improved communication, the status quo will continue to limit desired outcomes."

What is a model health care delivery system? "A system with adequate resources for all patients, regardless of their ability to pay; patients who will take responsibility for their care, and physicians who care and will partner with their patients to achieve better outcomes."

He believed that the "give and take of good communication" is the responsibility of both doctors and patients. "If patients and doctors don't commit to improved communication," he warned, "the *status quo* will continue to limit desired outcomes."

Patients as Patients

Subject: Male
Race: African American
Diagnosis: Bipolar disorder

This patient, currently a resident, under court supervision, in a halfway house for men addicted to alcohol or other drugs, was diagnosed as bipolar in 1996 and has been hospitalized 14 times since then for stays ranging from two weeks to nine months in private and state mental institutions. His diagnosis was based on his acting out in a disruptive behavior and was treated initially by a therapist without medication.

The patient reported an 18-month period without medication and without incident. When his physician became aware of the non-compliance, he insisted that the patient resume medication. In spite of complaints and requests of various physicians, he believes that he is continually overmedicated. He admits to moderate use of alcohol and marijuana, explaining that they stabilized his moods. Sleep deprivation causes him to become anxious, which results in readmission.

He finds it impossible to establish an on-going relationship with one physician because of the rotation of physicians in his clinic or hospital setting. "If the doctors listened to me," he says, "they would realize that I am a genius and very special, that my behavior is really not weird, just different. . . .I am manic more often than depressed, but sometimes my good moods look manic and everyone freaks."

His relationship with his family is also somewhat unstable: "My mother is afraid of me," he says. "She thinks my behavior is abnormal and sends me back to the doctors who treat me like a kid. Even so, I relate to my mother better than anyone. She is not afraid to show her love for me. My father is disappointed that I did not follow his footsteps into public life. I still love him and he loves me."

> "If I could change the health care system, I would make doctors listen and show more respect for mental patients. We have feelings, too."

The patient had many pertinent observations to make about the health care system and doctor-patient relationships. The following represents a sampling of them:

- Physicians give the patient the impression that they know all the answers related to the disease even when they do not.

- Physicians in outpatient settings give fewer medicines; those in inpatient facilities often over-medicate.

- Mental institutions focus on your mind and ignore the medical problems that may be the cause of strange behavior.

- Female physicians relate to patients better than male doctors do. They are more understanding, more sensitive, and less judgmental. They are willing to listen and treat you like a person, not just another patient.

Subject: **Male business executive**
Race: **African American**
Diagnosis: **Kidney transplant**

This patient, who described himself as a long-term end-stage renal disease patient with a kidney transplant of 12 years, spoke candidly about the problems he encountered in negotiating the worlds of primary care and nephrology.

"It is quite difficult to develop a relationship with your family doctor when you are in an on-going relationship with a nephrologist," the patient said. "Some primary care physicians are reluctant to refer to specialists; mine said he could handle my problem since it is 'only' maintenance." He also commented on the time constraints placed on doctor-patient relationships. "The doctor seems to take as little time as possible with the patient," he said. "I almost have to grab the doctor's arm to make him talk to me. Unless I am really sick, I don't bother him. They just want acute patients; chronic patients take too long."

He described the eight different medications he is required to take each day, remarking that his physicians had "glossed" over the many side effects of the various medicines. He said his anxiety as a patient is related to the frequent unexpected side effects of new medications.

He believes that patients and physicians should have a formal service agreement to spell out the terms of their partnership and that doctors "should learn to communicate

> **"Patients and physicians should have a formal service agreement to spell out the terms of their partnership."**

better with their long-term patients." He is particularly concerned by the cultural gaps and communication problems he has observed between African American patients and foreign-born physicians.

More than willing to assume responsibility for his own health, he stated, "If I don't agree with a doctors' instructions, I do not follow them. For example, my gout medication requires some adjustments by me because the doctor's instruction causes me to get sick. I process information and then make informed decisions on the treatment I will receive. I have become skilled in pain-management versus pill-management. I have to be proactive about my health in order to survive."

Subject: Male school teacher
Race: African American
Diagnosis: Multiple myeloma

This interview was conducted with the patient's wife after his death. The wife wanted to discuss the incredible strength displayed by her husband and the loving care he received from his many doctors and nurses.

The patient lived for four years after diagnosis of multiple myeloma. The diagnosis and search for a "cure" led the family to two out-of-state cities for extended periods of time. The physicians in each city were truthful about the slim possibility of survival. While they held out little hope, however, the physicians encouraged the patient to live each day to the fullest.

> "Physicians treated the family as an extension of the patient...and were always willing to answer questions."

The patient's wife expressed surprise at the outpouring of love from the physicians. They treated the family as an extension of the patient, and they were thoughtful and always willing to answer questions from the patient and from family members. At no time during her husband's illness, she said, was he made to feel as if he were a bother and or that he deserved anything less than the best medical care available.

She described her husband as valiant as he endured pain and the physical indignities of terminal illness. He served as a role model for his family and friends as he waited for death with quiet dignity and peace.

As evidence of the physicians' enduring love and concern for the whole family, she shared two letters, received after the patient's death, that diminished the weight of her grief:

From Physician A:
"Caring for the patient was a reminder to me that we physicians must learn not only to treat the terminal patient but also to provide comfort for the patient and his family. The patient faced the disease and the long fight with great dignity. He protected his family from his pain as one final declaration of his love. He was blessed to have his devoted family showing their eternal love at his side throughout his challenge." *[This physician and his wife attended the funeral and have kept in touch with the family.]*

From Physician B:
"I hope his last weeks were bearable and pain free during his last angry myeloma relapse. The patient was brave as he battled the disease; he was an example for us all. It was an honor to meet and treat such a brave man."

Subject: Retired professional football running back/business executive

Race: African American

Diagnosis: Rotator cuff repair

When this vice president of a multi-media corporation and former football pro, needed repair to his rotator cuff, he asked his former football associates for a referral to an orthopedic surgeon. He chose one that had been recommended by several former teammates.

On the basis of his experience, the patient discussed the importance of "before-hand" knowledge of physician expertise and patient relations skills. He made an effort to develop a relationship with the

> **Information on post-surgery pain and recovery was "too little, too late."**

surgeon prior to surgery and reported that the surgeon explained the surgery in great detail and answered the patient's questions with clarity. Information provided on post-surgery pain and recovery, however, he said, was "too little, too late." The physician failed to communicate the degree and severity of pain or the extreme physical limitations caused by the shoulder immobility.

His anticipated three-month rehabilitation extended to six months. This prolonged rehab caused great frustration because it impacted on his ability to work, which in turn caused an unanticipated financial hardship.

The patient contrasted the difference in how an athlete is treated as compared with a "normal patient" with a sports injury. Athletes are expected to play with pain and return to play quickly after surgery, and, he believed, physicians respond to team managers by returning the player to the field with great speed. "Normal" (non-athlete) patients seem to receive more consideration, he said.

The time he spends with his primary care physician, he reported, is determined by costs more than by regulations. "I think about my deductible and that drives the way I request doctor appointments. If the discomfort is bearable, I'll wait to call my doctor. I also let my body dictate the frequency of my physical therapy rather than the doctor's instruction."

When he does see the physician, he said, "I tell my doctor what I expect from him. Good communication is critical to maximizing my time spent with my doctor. Insurance company policies should include a mandatory training program to train physicians to communicate more effectively."

One reason for time constraints is the inefficiencies of the health care system, he believes. As an example, he detailed an experience in an urgi-care center, compared to visiting a barber. At the barbershop, he said, he went in, waited briefly (or not at all), was served promptly, and left 20 or 30 minutes later. In the urgi-care center, he entered the doctor's office, registered, waited, was taken to an exam room, waited and waited, a nurse took a history and vital signs, waited, waited, and waited, the doctor reviewed nurse's notes, asked a few questions, ordered tests, waited some more, tests were performed, waited again, and the doctor returned to announce, "There's nothing urgently wrong. Call your primary care physician in the A.M." Total time spent in the center: more than four hours.

"Sometimes," the patient observed, "it is easier, quicker, and more productive to go to the barber shop than to receive care in an urgi-care center."

Subject: **Waitress**
Race: **Caucasian**
Diagnosis: End Stage Renal Disease

This 37-year-old patient, who had experienced "poor health" since age 12, was diagnosed with kidney disease in 1994. Her family doctor encouraged her to continue working after her diagnosis and did not discuss the possibility of a transplant because she did well on dialysis and his attitude was "Why tamper with a good thing?"

For the patient, however, dialysis was not such a "good thing." She discussed at length her frustration with the dialysis routine and admitted that she was in denial for the first 18 months of her treatment. She was consistently non-compliant during that period, and the nephrologist seemed not to care. She sel-

> **Only a renal resident listened and heard this patient. "He's an example of old-fashioned doctoring."**

dom saw him in the dialysis facility, getting instructions only through the renal nurse.

Her non-compliance led to three hospitalizations. During each treatment and hospitalization, the patient said she tried to discuss her finances and the difficulty she had in maintaining a renal diet within her limited budget. "No one listened," she said, until she met with "a nice young nephrology resident." Unlike the other doctors, he treated her like a person instead of a renal patient, she said, and in words she understood, he explained the consequences of non-compliance. He arranged dietician consults and asked the renal social worker to help her to find some source of supplemental income. The resident, she said, was an example of "old-fashioned doctoring."

The patient states that she is now compliant and hopes for a transplant.

Subject: **Male Internal Revenue agent**
Race: **Caucasian**
Diagnosis: Coronary Heart Disease

When this 57-year-old patient was diagnosed with coronary heart disease in 1990, the diagnosis entailed major modifications to his life style of travel and sports activity.

The patient is grateful to both his primary care physician and his cardiologist for their supportiveness. They encouraged him to learn about his disease and referred him to a nutritionist and, due to the nature of his work, to a stress management counselor. The patient's employer displayed great sensitivity to his need to "slow down," relieving him of the need to travel extensively on the job.

> "I am a full partner in the development of my care plans. When I disagree, I am heard."

The patient admitted that he was slow to learn the value of asking questions when he did not understand the information presented by the physicians, but, he said, "I am now a full partner with my doctors in the development of my care plans. When I disagree, I am heard, and plans are sometimes modified. It is good to be alive. I am thankful for the wonderful doctors who take good care of me."

Subject: **Retired businessman**
Race: **Caucasian**
Diagnosis: **Coronary Heart Disease**

Diagnosed with coronary heart disease at age 57, the patient has been under treatment for eight years. The severity of the illness and the high stress associated with his business caused him to retire early.

"I used to give orders. Now I take them—from my doctor," he remarked wryly. He drew a sharply contrasting picture of his primary care physician and his cardiologist. The primary care

> "Doctor's effort to calm me down is a day late and a dollar short."

physician, who is an old friend, engages him in cordial give and take as they discuss health issues. "He listens most of the time," the patient says. "I hear him sometimes."

With the cardiologist, it is a different story. The cardiologist, whom he calls "Dr. Doorknob," stands at the door after his examination, reports the exam findings (sometimes not good), and then says, "we'll discuss this next week." The patient described his anxiety and frustration at having no opportunity to ask questions or address his concerns until the next visit at which time the physician may try to allay his fears and prescribe new medication. At this point, he said, "the doctor's effort to calm me down is a day late and a dollar short."

Subject: **Male restaurateur and decorated veteran**
Race: **Caucasian**
Diagnosis: End-Stage Renal Disease

This 81-year-old owner of a family-owned, upscale restaurant led an exciting life before poor health forced him into semi-retirement. A college graduate, he attained the rank of Colonel in the U. S. Army during World War II and participated in the allied liberation of Belgium and the Battle of the Bulge. His combat experience earned him a Purple Heart with clusters, a Bronze Star, a Combat Infantry Badge, a recommendation for the Silver Star, and honors in the Officers' Candidate School Hall of Fame at Fort Benning, GA. As an octogenarian, he viewed his end-

stage renal disease as simply an "inconvenience," and he contin-
ued to direct the family business from his wheel chair, greeting
and visiting with patrons as they entered the restaurant.

The author was privileged to observe this patient in several roles over the course of 18 months:

- As a doting father and grandfather who worked very
  hard to shield his family from his pain and discomfort.

- As a dialysis patient who remained humble in his relationships with other patients and the staff at the dialysis
  unit, neither expecting nor seeking special treatment

  > "With my faith in God, a family who loves and supports me, and caring and competent physicians, I am not afraid. I can manage anything."

  because of his position in the community. He treated the
  staff with great courtesy, often voicing his appreciation
  for their care. By his choice, few of the other patients
  knew of his celebrity. Nevertheless, they appreciated his
  encouragement to follow the doctor's instructions and to
  live life fully each day.

- As a true partner with his physicians in the course of his
  treatment. He considered his doctors to be open and
  honest: "They tell me what I need to know and accept
  my decisions regarding my care," he said.

Was he angry because his illness had changed his life?
"No," he said, explaining that "I've had a beautiful life,

more good days than bad days. With my faith in God, a family who loves and supports me, and caring and competent physicians, I am not afraid. I can manage anything."

He saw his nephrologist as a sensitive friend and a great doctor who would do all that was "feasible" for a man in his condition. . "He discusses renal disease and its prognosis with me and my family in words we can understand. Other doctors could learn much about talking to patients by observing my doctor in action."

The patient died in March 2003. His nephrologist died six months later, in September 2003.

Barriers to Communication —and Care

6

I wish my doctor would stop changing my medicines as often as he changes his ties. It is very expensive.

(Patient)

Some patients withhold personal information that affects their health and well-being. They should be more honest about their lifestyles and about therapies they disagree with or don't like rather than not complying.

(Doctor)

Webster defines a barrier as "anything that obstructs progress, access, etc."[5] Throughout our dialogue via the survey, focus groups, and interviews, physicians and patients identified both external and internal barriers that impact negatively on communication and, ultimately, on the delivery and receipt of quality health care. Access to care is severely compromised when health care providers fail to tell and patients fail to ask how to enter and negotiate the system, and the quality of care as well as outcomes are diminished when patients fail to say (and their physicians fail to hear) their reasons for not complying with medical instruction.

Physician-Identified Barriers

Regulations from state and federal agencies and third party payers were at the top of the physicians' list of barriers to doctor/patient communication. Insurance company paperwork, often redundant, and dictates as to the amount of time to be spent per office visit, doctors said, reduced their time with patients and, consequently, the time for questions, information sharing, and establishing a trusting relationship. At the same time, they felt that governmental and insurance guidelines interfere with the doctor's ability to diagnose and treat patients, with their decisions overturned by "second-guessing" and denial of claims. A number of physicians pointed out that inadequate insurance payments and "exorbitant" malpractice premiums place a financial hardship on physicians, forcing them to see more patients in order to pay the bills.

Patients came in for a share of the blame, too. Patients sometimes withhold pertinent information that is critical to an accurate diagnosis, doctors reported. They also stressed that patients often lack the background or education to understand the ramifications of their diagnosis and the importance of immediate life-style changes, such as weight loss or smoking cessation. This lack of understanding is compounded by patients' tendency to compare symptoms and diagnoses with friends and family members with the expectation of similar outcomes—and by the lack of a family support system, in many cases, to reinforce the need for life-style changes.

Patient-Identified Barriers

Not surprisingly, patients had their own concerns about such issues as time, costs, and psychosocial factors, but their view differed significantly from that expressed by the physicians. Most patients placed a high priority on having adequate time with their physicians to discuss medical problems and to ask questions, and they believed that this is often lacking because of over-scheduling ("Too many patients scheduled at the same time!") and results in long waiting times. Most office hours, they pointed out, do not accommodate the needs of working patients and may cause patients to delay seeking care because they must miss work to see the doctor.

To patients who lack adequate insurance coverage, costs are a major barrier to accessing care and complying with treatment regimens. Paying for prescription drugs is a serious burden for many patients, who confessed that they sometimes reduce the dosage or use drugs selectively to save money. They faulted physicians for not distributing samples more generously, especially when a new medication is prescribed and the patient's tolerance for it is not yet determined. Non-compliance with dietary recommendations was often based on financial considerations as well as cultural concerns and preferences.

Psychosocial concerns, however, were paramount in the patients' minds. Many felt that physicians lack respect for patients' intelligence and show irritation or anger when they ask questions or disagree with the doctor ("When I disagree with the doctor, it is easier not to follow his instructions than to argue—he thinks my brain is the size of a pea.") One patient reported that his doctor objected to the patient's wife accompanying him to an office visit. "He says she interferes," he noted, "but I say she helps me to understand." Another complained that her doctor doesn't listen to her concerns and "gets mad" when she asks questions. "As a result," she said, "I don't trust his instructions."

The Impact of Ethnicity

Ethnicity was found to present barriers to the seeking of care, provision of care, and the outcome of treatments. Patients, in particular, cited "cultural differences" as the source of many problems in communication with "clinic doctors," whose foreign accents created a serious language barrier. When they complained, patients reported, they were "ignored" or told that the physician was competent and that the accent was not a problem.

Patients commented on the rigid refusal of physicians to listen to their concerns. Patients found foreign-born physicians were often "stand-offish" and unwilling to enter into social conversations. They believed a definite "caste" system was operating, with patients looked upon as diseases rather than as people.

Cultural differences were blamed for much patient noncompliance, particularly with dietary restrictions. Patients believed that physicians should instruct dieticians to work with them to incorporate cultural eating patterns and preferences in designing therapeutic diets. Physicians and dieticians should also consider the patient's financial situation before ordering diets that may impose a hardship on the family by requiring special foods or supplements that are costly.

Most physicians in the focus groups and interviews discounted the complaints, and those who were foreign-born protested, "My colleagues understand me. Why can't my patients?" Many physicians did not understand the need for social discourse or why its lack was identified as a barrier by some patients. The physicians were emphatic in their statements: "I am their doctor, not their friend." Others expressed frustration with their patients' lack of "gratitude" for the available health care services. Many blamed noncompliance on the patients' unwillingness to make life style changes "because they don't care" or because they don't understand the seriousness of their illness.

National origin, however, was not the only source of cultural differences. A number of African American patients commented on their interactions with Caucasian doctors who, the patients said, conveyed the attitude that "You cause your problems because of your chosen life style so stop complaining!" Patients perceived that the same racism they experience in the "outside" world is alive and well and thriving in many clinic settings.

An article on the Virginia Polytechnic Institute's web site, "Culture-Sensitive Health Care"[2] offers the following recommendations for a good professional relationship with African American patients:

1. **Don't assume.** Many African Americans will be similar in background to the caregiver, and many will be of different backgrounds. Whatever the race of the caregiver, no assumption should be made about the similarity or differ-

ence in background between caregiver and patient. With respect to health-related beliefs and practices, an African American patient may be as different from an African American caregiver as from a White, Hispanic, or Asian physician. On the other hand, an African American patient may be quite similar to the caregiver, regardless of the caregiver's race. It is the task of the caregiver to probe and listen carefully to the patient to determine the patient's expectations and beliefs.

2. Ask for causes. When taking the initial history and performing a physical examination, ask patients not only about their symptoms but also whether they know what caused the illness. Patients' answers may reveal whether they subscribe to a folk or magical belief system.

3. Listen without judgment. It is essential during all stages of a consultation that the caregiver listen carefully and sympathetically. Refrain from expressing anything that might be interpreted as judgmental, patronizing, or ridiculing.

Doctors tend to underestimate patients' desire for information and to misperceive the process of information giving. Doctors' nonverbal communication abilities are associated with outcomes in medical care such as satisfaction and compliance.

Physicians who have themselves been patients remarked in focus groups and in interviews on how their own experiences had heightened their awareness in terms of sensitivity and the need for clarity as they spoke to their patients. Their comments echoed this humble statement by Michael LaCombe, MD, who wrote a book entitled *On Being a Doctor:*

> It has now been three years since diagnosis. All post-procedural examinations have been within normal limits. I was given the unique opportunity to see life from various extremes. Being a patient was terribly unpleasant. I know how my patients feel. I know that there is much more to being a good physician than just being a good diagnostician. I have learned empathy and compassion. Facing death itself produced an awareness of my own mortality I will never forget.[6]

Expectations vs. Assumptions | 7

Expectations and assumptions must be communicated by physicians and patients. Non-communicated assumptions and expectations result in dissatisfaction in both parties.

(Doctor)

I really am always having trouble with blood pressure medications. My doctor thinks I'm not taking them, but I am— as directed!

(Patient)

An *expectation*, according to Webster[5], is the prospect of future benefit, and an *assumption*, something taken for granted. Good communication is based on shared expectations and common assumptions, but—as the survey, focus groups, and interviews revealed—doctors and patients generally are *not* on the same page. Therein lies the source of many of the communication problems they experience.

Physicians *expected* patients to come to them for care because the patients *assumed* the physician is competent and able to address their illness. Physicians *assume* the patient will follow instructions without question or challenge while patients often *expect* the physician to answer questions (even if they weren't asked) and to negotiate a treatment regimen with positive results. These assumptions and expectations result in communication issues.

Neither patient nor physician has verbalized expectations or assumptions. It is assumed that each knows intuitively what is expected and assumed.

Following are some common expectations and assumptions that resulted in the breakdown of communication between doctor and patient:

Patients *expected* physicians to be available when needed and to provide adequate time for patients to share their concerns. Physicians *assumed* that patients understood the variety of demands on their availability and time. Neither partner shared their *expectations* or *assumptions*.

Physicians *expected* patients to follow their instruction relative to compliance (i.e., diet, life-style changes). Patients *assumed* that physicians would understand the psychosocial impediments that delayed or precluded compliance. Physicians *assumed* that their office hours were reasonable, while patients *expected* greater flexibility to accommodate employment schedules or childcare needs.

Patients *expected* to have their physician answer all their questions personally while physicians *assumed* that patients understand that the use of physician-extenders (persons trained and certified to perform many clinical procedures under the supervision of a physician) is an effort to be more available. In fact, patients view the practice as evasive and unsatisfactory.

Physicians *assumed* that patients understand the information given to them. Patients *expected* doctors to take the time to explain things fully and in language they can understand.

Patients *expected* to be seen promptly in the doctor's office. When delays occur, physicians *assumed* that patients knew that unforeseen problems had caused the schedule problems.

Physicians *expected* to share news, "good or bad," with patients as quickly as possible. Patients *assumed* that the physician knows how much information the patient can handle and will handle bad news delicately.

Physicians *assumed* non-compliance on the basis of clinical indicators such as elevated blood pressure or failure to lose weight. Patients *expected* physicians to believe them when they describe their efforts to follow the doctor's instructions.

Physicians often *assumed* the patient is not as ill as he thinks he is, based on the reported symptoms. Patients *expected* physicians to listen to the symptom report with an open mind, focusing on individual patient concerns.

Patients *assumed* that physicians can make adequate diagnoses by telephone. Physicians *expected* to see patients in a follow-up visit as soon as possible after telephone consultation.

Physicians *assumed* that patients will disclose all information pertinent to a final diagnosis. Patients *expected* to share physical symptoms but often declined to disclose "personal" information.

What does the patient want from the physician encounter? That question is easier to ask than to answer. In the words of one physician, "they (patients) want to be able to trust the competence and efficacy of their caregivers. They want to be able to negotiate the health care system effectively and to be treated with dignity and respect. Patients want to understand how their sickness or treatment will affect their lives, and they often fear that their doctors are not telling them everything they need to know. Patients worry about and want to learn how to care for themselves away from the clinical setting. They want us to focus on their pain, physical discomfort, and functional disabilities. They want to discuss the effect their illness will have on their family, friends, and finances. And they worry about the future."

Where is the "Me" in Your "We"?

My doctor takes things that I talk to him about so lightly-as if I didn't know what was going on with my illness.

(Patient)

It is important to base expectations for participation in the care plan on the patients' intellectual and emotional ability to do so.

(Doctor)

By definition, partnership recognizes the "me" in "we" statements: Webster points out that being a partner implies "participation, association, and joint interest."[9] The physician/patient partnerships that were observed or reported by our participants, however, existed more often on paper than in practice. The "joint interest" in the definition implies that in successful partnerships, both partners benefit from the relationship: physicians benefit from the tangible and intangible rewards of using their medical training to provide quality health care, and patients benefit from access to medical expertise, with the expectation of beneficial outcomes.

To the patients in the surveys, focus groups, and interviews, their "participation" in the various options related to their treatment regimen was minimal. With few opportunities to discuss their own preferences with the physician before the plan was finalized, they commented wryly on the physician's frequent use of "we" as he/she described a proposed treatment plan. Too often, patients believed, decisions are made for them without their participation. Physicians who impose diets, life-style changes, and medications frequently fail to realize the importance of patient input and "buy-in" to such decisions. A special diet may present financial hardship for patients of limited means, particularly when it involves preparing separate menus for the patient and for the rest of the family. Similarly, some diet changes conflict with cultural food patterns and preferences. Discussing the issues with the patient may lead to strategies for modifying the family diet to address the special needs of the patient or adapting a new diet to traditional food preferences. Absence of sensitivity to patient needs and preferences almost guarantees non-compliance.

When physicians order major changes in life-style, they must realize that unhealthy habits are learned behavior and they can be changed or modified only with new learned behaviors. Patients must be patiently educated to the benefits of life-style changes and the consequences of non-compliant behaviors. Patients should not be judged but rather encouraged to embrace the recommended changes for life's sake.

Physicians have the responsibility to discuss possible side effects of medications so that patients are prepared for them. They should also be sensitive to the financial burden that medications can place on patients without prescription drug coverage and, when possible, use professional samples to introduce new medications rather than committing the patient to the cost of a month's supply of a drug that may not be tolerated well.

Much time in the discussion of the "new medicine" is dedicated to the concept of a partnership between physicians and patients. Both partners must be committed to the give and take of such a relationship and willing to be patient with each other in order to make the partnership a reality and achieve a positive outcome.

Courtesy Is Contagious

The Bible warns, "Be not deceived: evil communications corrupt good manners." (Corinthians 15:33). The reverse is also true. Both physicians and patients remarked on the lack of common courtesy they experience in health care encounters and suggested that such thoughtlessness and insensitivity could undermine doctor-patient communication. Both parties admitted that their reaction to discourtesy was to respond in kind.

Patients resented the long waits in the doctor's office and poor scheduling in clinics as a statement of the professionals' disregard for patients' time and convenience. Many complained of "rudeness" on the part of the office staff. They were especially critical of what they saw as the physician's attitude of superiority ("He talks down to me and uses words I don't understand") and resented the fact that the doctor expects to be addressed as "Doctor" but routinely calls patients by their first names. Patients also cited physician insensitivity to their need for privacy by talking loud enough for patients in adjoining cubicles to overhear.

Physicians presented their own list of complaints about patients who are chronically late, rude to the clerical staff, or expect to be seen before their scheduled appointment. They also cited patients who "challenged the doctor's credentials" by disagreeing with recommended treatments and those who withhold information that is crucial to accurate diagnoses.

Patients and physicians agreed that neither apologizes for lateness and seldom utters a simple "Thank you." All agreed that courtesy is contagious.

In Their Own Words

My doctor looks into my soul and helps me make it through the day.

(Patient)

My patient wants to learn about his disease, and I want to teach him. How cool is that?

(Doctor)

Patients and physicians who participated in the study were asked to contribute to a "wish list" that would create the optimum components for improved doctor/patient communication and relationships. Each was asked simply to complete two sentences:

"I wish my doctor (or patient) would . . . ." and

"I wish my doctor (or patient) would *not*. . . . ."

Both groups exhibited some hesitation initially, suggesting perhaps that they felt that the *status quo* of poor communication would persist, regardless of their input. Many said that the ability to make meaningful changes was out of their control, and some hesitated to speak out for fear of offending the individual (doctor or patient) whose behavior was questionable. Most did respond to the questions, however. While the initial survey results separated the comments of renal and multi-diagnosis patients and those of nephrologists and other specialties, the similarity among the groups was so striking that, in the final analysis, the lists were combined except when references applied specifically to patients on dialysis. In some cases, disease-specific references are included.

Among the perceptions common across the board: Patients regretted the absence of greater personal interaction and resented being treated "as a disease, not as a person." Physicians felt that their competency was challenged by aggressive patient questioning. Both physicians and patients acknowledged the urgent need to improve communication and decried the lack of courtesy, sensitivity, and willingness to share information.

Here, in their own words, are the suggestions doctors and patients have for each other: their prescriptions for improving communication:

From patients:

On Availability

I wish my doctor WOULD:

- Have office hours more often and longer.
- Provide more flexible office hours and rounds for people who work.
- Be more available to talk to me. Sometimes I call after office hours, and he gets annoyed with me.
- See me more often than once a month.
- See me sooner when I have a new problem.
- Give some good attention.

- Provide the quality of care that Medicare requires and pays for. The short visits and unavailability do not provide quality.
- Make more rounds.
- Stop by the clinic when he has time to see patients and not just review charts.

I wish my doctor would NOT:

- Over-schedule patients, so that the waiting room is not packed and you don't have to wait so long.
- Have such a large caseload.
- Make patients wait so long in the waiting room.
- Leave the facility so quickly.
- Interrupt me when I try to tell him something.

On Communication

I wish my doctor WOULD:

- Consider and discuss side effects of medications before I buy medicine that I can't tolerate.
- Spend more time talking to me instead of sending messages to me by the nurse.
- Tell me the truth.
- Remember he is talking to a patient and not another doctor—use words that I understand.
- Understand that I am really trying to follow his instructions even if the lab results are not good.
- Speak English better. Sometimes I say yes when I really don't understand the question or the instructions.
- Let me finish my complaints before he tells me that's expected because of the disease.

- Understand that I don't lie about my compliance.
- Listen more.
- Keep me more informed of my progress and problems.
- Hear and not just listen; help and not just answer.

I wish my doctor would NOT:

- Fail to follow-up when he changes my medication.
- Just shake hands and run off to visit other patients. He should at least ask me how I feel.
- Put me in the hospital for every little thing.
- Interrupt me when I talk to him.
- Prescribe medications for every problem.
- Assume I understand medical talk.
- Withhold information related to the deterioration of my condition.
- Work on a "need to know" basis.
- Give vague answers to my questions and then get mad when I push for better answers.
- Talk "down" to me.
- Speak English with such a thick foreign accent.
- Talk too much rather than listening to me more.
- Make snap judgments about my medicine dosage. It keeps changing, and that's very expensive.

On Courtesy

I wish my doctor WOULD:

- Ask his office staff to be more courteous to me when I call his office.
- Tell office staff what they should or should not say to patients. They need to be more polite.

- Treat my wife with more courtesy. He does not like her to ask questions about my care.
- Return my phone calls within a reasonable time (i.e., within twenty-four hours).

I wish my doctor would NOT:

- Refuse to return my phone calls.
- Interrupt me when I try to tell him something.
- Yell at me as though I am stupid and then rush to see the next patient.
- Make patients wait so long in the waiting room.
- Exhibit such a condescending attitude toward my family and me.
- Give me a hard time for calling with a "simple complaint." How am I supposed to know what is serious?
- Ignore complaints from patients until they become emergencies.

On Quality Time

I wish my doctor WOULD:

- "Hold" his calls unless there is an emergency so that he can focus on me.
- Allow more time during the appointment for patients to tell their problems.
- Sit down and talk and listen to me.
- Spend more time with me so that I can share my concerns.
- Spend more time visiting each patient at the clinic.
- Be able to give the care and individual attention to each of his patients that they need and he quite obviously would desire for himself.

- Pay a little more attention to my needs.
- Take more time with me and really look into things that I bring to his attention about the unit and staff.
- Take the time to check my meds more often.
- Slow down and spend more time with me.
- Be able to discuss with me my frustrations with regard to the many restrictions that I face.
- Schedule quarterly appointments with family members to discuss my condition.
- Allow more time to discuss my concerns as a patient.

I wish my doctor would NOT:

- Always hurry through my visit, just like an assembly line.
- Hurry through patient-doctor treatment/interviews.
- Hurry through my examination and explanation of my lab values.

On Sensitivity

I wish my doctor WOULD:

- Be more sensitive when he has to tell me "bad" news. "Don't be such a baby!" is not what I need to hear.
- Take me at my appointed time and not make me wait so very long. When you are sick, the waiting time seems much longer.
- Show more interest in me as a person instead of acting like I am a medical record.
- Show more concern and act as though I was someone he wanted to help.
- Be more attentive, responsive, and creative in my care.
- Ask me about my life-style and family.

- Listen to my feelings and be more considerate of my age—I don't like "off-color" jokes.
- Shorten the waiting time in his office.
- Be more attentive, responsive, and creative in addressing my progress.
- Show more concern and act as though he wanted to help my mother. The doctors always made it seem like it was a chore to take care of my mother.
- Listen to me.
- Take care of my pain when I say I am in pain.
- Talk to me, as he would want someone to talk to him.
- Understand that I did not go to medical school so I don't know enough not to worry.
- Talk to me instead of my mother. I'm 16. I can understand his comments.
- Be a little more people oriented. Try to converse with us more. Make us feel like people, not just patients.
- Stop changing my medicines as often as he changes his ties. It is very expensive.
- Stop passing patients around in his group with little or no information.
- Just ask me how I'm doing instead of telling me what the nurse said about my condition.

I wish my doctor would NOT:

- Judge me for my life-style and treat me as if I don't deserve his time.
- Treat me like I have no brain.
- Give special treatment to his favorite patients (i.e., slip them through the side door)

- Use me as a "guinea pig" for the new doctors (residents).
- Take things that I talk to him about so lightly as if I didn't know what was going on with my illness.
- Have partners that don't know my case.
- Yell at me as though I was stupid and then rush to see the next patient.
- Give certain patients special treatment.
- Rush off when he doesn't want to hear what I have to say.
- Treat me like I have no brain.
- Forget me.
- Become annoyed with me because I can't tell indigestion from a heart attack.
- Compare me with his other patients. I am an individual. He needs to recognize that and treat me accordingly.
- Question my description of my symptoms (i.e., "You really are not as sick as you think you are.")

On Respect

I wish my doctor WOULD:

- Slow down and show me a little respect.
- Return phone calls more promptly.
- Respect my privacy.
- Believe me: I really am always having trouble with blood pressure medications. He thinks I'm not taking them, but I am—as directed!

I wish my doctor would NOT:

- Interrupt me when I try to tell him something.

On Responsiveness

I wish my doctor WOULD:

- Answer my questions completely, not half answer the question.
- Consult with my other doctors to arrive at the best overall treatment plan for me.
- Address my notes the day I send them in with my mother, the patient. He told me to do this, and as yet (in 5 weeks) we have not properly communicated effectively.
- Cure me!

I wish my doctor would NOT:

- Try different drugs for high blood pressure until one drug works. He should be able to come up with a series of meds that work that don't have so many bad side effects.
- Put me off when I ask hard questions.
- Just listen and make no comment.

Miscellaneous

I wish my doctor WOULD:

- Consider holistic medicine to help improve my conditions.
- Slow down—he is going to burn out.

I wish my doctor would NOT:

- Charge me for every single visit. Sometimes they do not do anything but ask me questions—no exams—just another prescription, but still I'm charged the same as when he really examines me.

- Put interns in charge of my care. Does Medicare pay less for intern care?
- Have to be responsible for a large patient load.

Dialysis Patients:

Dialysis patients shared many concerns with the multi-diagnosis patients, but some comments relate specifically to the dialysis experience:

Dialysis patients wished their renal doctors WOULD:

- Be more available at treatment times.
- Visit the dialysis unit more often.
- Be available for all shifts at dialysis. There are times when the group rounds in the morning, and I arrive in the afternoon. This makes it impossible to discuss my concerns. They should alternate times.
- Have the courtesy to answer my questions. I just started on dialysis and never knew anything about kidney failure. He has to explain everything to me. I am 57 years old and scared to death.
- Have told me about what my quality of life would be six or seven years after starting dialysis (sexual function performance, etc.)
- Reduce my dialysis time from four to three hours. I feel better with three hours.
- Give me an overall evaluation of my progress on dialysis on a regular basis.
- Include other members of the transplant team in discussing patient treatment options.

- Give all patients a turn at being first to be hooked up to the machine.
- Give me more advice to help me cope with dialysis and all the meds I have to take.
- Be more aggressive in monitoring my chances to receive a transplant.
- Track my waiting time to receive a new kidney.
- Be more considerate if we have problems maintaining our dry weight.
- Help me more with my kidneys and my cancer.
- Pull a kidney out of her pocket.
- Ignore Medicare guideline for epogen use; I want to feel good all the time.
- Heal my kidney disease.
- Invent a reliable artificial kidney—I would be a guinea pig for him.

Dialysis patients wished their renal doctors would NOT:

- Increase my dialysis time based on one set of lab values.
- Ask so many questions about other people in the dialysis unit.
- Send his assistants to see me on dialysis. They don't care about me the way he does.
- Wake me when I'm asleep.
- Encourage me to have a transplant. (The first two failed.)
- Take my hope away. Without hope, there is no reason to get up in the morning.
- Keep saying "Are you sure I am one of your kidney doctors?" By now, he should know me.

From physicians:

On Compliance

I wish my patients WOULD:

- Take my medication as prescribed.
- Understand that compliance is an everyday adventure, not something to do when it is convenient.
- Keep appointments as scheduled.
- Become an active partner in the development of the treatment plan.
- Quit smoking!!!
- Be more compliant.
- Follow my instruction.
- Listen attentively and follow instruction.
- Understand how much their well-being is dependent on their action and lifestyle changes.

I wish my patients would NOT:

- Stop medication and not tell me.
- Miss appointments.
- Forget or neglect to call with problems.
- Become couch potatoes.
- Give up.

On Communication

I wish my patients WOULD:

- Tell me the truth about the symptoms they experience.
- Tell me if they don't understand my instructions.
- Talk to me as well as listen to me.

- Allow my partners to care for him in my absence. We are all equally competent to care for him.
- Learn the names, doses, and the reason for each medication and bring them for each appointment.
- Stop repeating information (inaccurate) gathered from newspapers or news programs.
- Be more interactive and respond to questions related to medication.
- Speak up when they don't understand all aspects of their medical management.
- Be more honest about which therapies they disagree with or don't like rather than not comply.
- Put a higher priority on their health.

I wish my patients would NOT:

- Blame me if the prognosis is not favorable.
- Demand treatment based on what their neighbors, friends, TV, or their mothers tell them.
- Withhold personal information that affects health and well-being.
- Come to see me but not value my opinion.
- Discuss their medical problems with non-medical people and judge the appropriateness of my advice regarding their care and treatment on the basis of what they say.

On Barriers to Care

I wish my patients WOULD:

- Take responsibility for the illness and do their part to improve the condition if possible or at least not make it worse.

- Learn about the disease to enhance understanding of the treatment plan and their need to participate in the plan.
- Take more responsibility for their health maintenance.

I wish my patients would NOT:

- Wait until they are urgent to call me.
- Allow adult children to interfere with their care when the child lives out of town or hasn't spoken with me.
- Fear health care as more likely to injure than to help them.
- Seek treatment over the telephone.
- Become depressed and give up.
- Blame other people for their medical condition instead of taking responsibility for their well-being.
- Ignore my instructions if they interfere with his/her lifestyle.
- Ask other patients for advice on health problems.
- Discount my advice.

On Courtesy

I wish my patients WOULD:

- Be more pleasant to my staff.

I wish my patients would NOT:

- Call after hours with very trivial complaints.
- Call after hours unless it's an emergency.
- Be so demanding and unappreciative of staff.

On Insurance/Government Guidelines

I wish my patients WOULD:

- Accept my treatment limitations dictated by their insurance carriers.
- Have better prescription drug coverage.

I wish my patients would NOT:

- Ask for a 90-day prescription for drugs that are not maintenance so they can save money.

Nephrologists:

In addition to echoing many of the comments above, nephrologists expressed concerns related specifically to patients on dialysis.

Nephrologists wished that their patients WOULD:

- Stay for their full treatment.
- Stick to their diet.
- Take medications as prescribed.
- Learn about their renal disease.
- Consider transplantation.
- Understand long-term implications of ESRD.
- Have their AV access inserted sooner.
- Take more initiative for their care.
- Call earlier with problems.
- Trust me and not take their anger out on me.

They wished that their patients would NOT:

- Miss appointments in my office.
- Skip treatments.
- Expect improvement in his condition without following my instructions.
- Lie to me about compliance. I read the lab results.
- Eat food so high in phosphorus.
- Miss dialysis treatments.
- Sign off early from dialysis.
- Ignore dietary consultation.
- Smoke or drink alcohol.
- Refuse to deal with other physicians in their physician's absence.
- Challenge the doctor's advice.
- Forget or neglect to call with problems.
- Become upset with other people and take it out on me.
- Take for granted that medicine will fix everything.
- Minimize condition changes.
- Say they understand when it is obvious they do not understand.
- Compare illnesses and symptoms with other patients.
- Take illegal drugs.
- Act as if their renal disease is the doctor's fault.
- Blow off the doctor's advice.
- Think dialysis is a punishment.
- Live their lives simply as dialysis patients.
- Be reluctant to take an active part in their treatment plan.
- Gain weight between treatments and lie about fluid intake.
- Focus on peripheral issues rather than central illnesses (e.g.,. mild edema rather than uncontrolled hypertension).
- Be rude to the doctor or the dialysis staff.

- Scare the dialysis staff with their abusive behavior.
- Be abusive to dialysis staff.
- Be referred late by the primary care physician and expect positive results.
- Have to wait so long for transplant evaluations.
- Ask the doctor to ignore Medicare guideline for EPO and prescribe it.

What's Right About Doctor-Patient Relationships

As instructive as the preceding "wishes" may be, perhaps the most dramatic guidance comes from the spontaneous praise expressed by doctors and patients about each other. Some, obviously, are on target and communicating well.

Here's what some patient respondents had to say about their physicians:

Patients said:

"My doctor is responsive to me, not reactionary."

"My doctor does fine by me."

"Doctor, please continue the good job!"

"I have no problems *at all* with my doctor. He is the best doctor I have ever had."

"My doctor stays the same. I have had several in the past but none as good as the one I have now."

"My doctor is special. He's first-class.

"My doctor is very good. I have no complaints."

"Doctor, stay as perfect as you are."

"Dr. S _____ is the best doctor any patient could wish for. May he live forever and may I never die."

"My doctor treats me with great respect—and I love him for it."

"My doctor treats me like a person."

"My doctor and I are equal partners."

"Me and my doctor are a team. We take good care of me."

"My doctor puts himself in my place and shows me the love and caring I need."

"My doctor always takes time to listen to me. Sometimes, he even agrees with me."

"My doctor does a lot for me. He really cares about my family and me."

"My doctors don't know how much I love them. They keep me alive."

"My doctor is a savior. He makes my life worth living."

"My doctor looks into my soul and helps me make it through the day."

Physicians said:

"I love patients who love themselves enough to take care of themselves."

"This patient makes my training worthwhile."

"My patients participate in their treatments."

"Families who support their patient are God-sent."

"I love it when my patients listen to my questions and respond with honest answers."

"My patients trust me—what an awesome responsibility!"

"When my patients take my advice and improve, they make me smile."

"My patient wants to learn about his disease, and I want to teach him. How cool is that?"

"My patient treats me with respect, and I return the favor."

"I wish I had a magic wand to cure illness. My patients don't deserve to suffer."

Prescription for Progress

I have become skilled in pain management versus pill management by listening to myself. I believe doctors should learn to communicate better with their patients. I have to be proactive about my health in order to survive.

(Patient)

Patients should take responsibility for learning about their illness and do their part to improve the condition if possible or at least not make it worse.

(Doctor)

The preceding chapters have identified many successes and failures as physicians and patients have attempted to fashion improved communication strategies. The problem of ineffective communication is solvable: there is an urgent need to execute a viable action plan. We are able to improve issues of poor communication if both parties—physicians and patients—commit to own responsibility for their roles in a successful relationship.

Both partners must critique their own behaviors and identify areas that need improvement. Language barriers were identified by many patients. For example, physicians who speak with foreign accents must acknowledge the difficulty that some patients have in understanding important information. These physicians must make every effort to ensure that patients understand them. By the same token, patients who speak with foreign accents or regional dialects must make similar efforts to ensure physician understanding. Gaps in comprehension may lead to wrong diagnoses, medication errors, and inaccurate instructions.

A conscious effort to identify components of effective communication will set the stage for improved dialogue. The sample communication contracts on the next two pages offer a model for patients and physicians to follow. Although I realize that most physicians will not actually implement the signed contracts, displaying them in the waiting room or making copies available to patients can serve as a constant reminder of the need for both doctors and patients to focus on clarifying their roles and responsibilities in the partnership.

Reproduction of the Patient and Physician Contracts and the Medical History Card on page 120 for personal or intra-office use is permitted by the author. These forms may not be reproduced in other publications or for sale without the author's written permission.

A Patient's Contract for Effective Communication

I promise to become a full partner with my physician in the management of my illness.

I promise to speak to my doctor in the same tone of respect that I expect.

I promise to prepare for my visit with a written list of my concerns so that I can maximize the time I spend with my doctor.

I promise to recognize my doctors' busy schedule and arrange a time to speak that is mutually convenient in non-emergency situations.

I promise to keep scheduled appointments on time or telephone my doctor's office to cancel and reschedule.

I promise to show the same courtesy that I expect to receive.

I promise to take responsibility to learn about my illness and to ask questions to improve my understanding.

I promise not to withhold information from my doctor that may affect a suggested treatment plan.

I promise to discuss with my doctor any situations that will prevent me from following the recommendations or medications prescribed.

I promise to make my health a priority.

I understand that this relationship may be terminated if my doctor and I are unable to communicate to ensure the provision of the best medical care.

_____

Patient's Signature

_____

Date   Physician's Signature

© 2003 by Margaret Smith Washington

A Physician's Contract for Effective Communication

I promise to acknowledge my patient as a full partner in the development of a treatment plan in the management of illness.

I promise to speak to my patient in language that is clear, concise, and not patronizing.

I promise to speak to my patient in a tone of respect that acknowledges my patient's adult or youth status.

I promise to make myself available for a reasonable period of time to listen to patient concerns and to clarify information that my patient did not understand.

I promise to be sensitive to my patients' time and have appointments scheduled with a reasonable expectation of staying on schedule.

I promise to show my patient the same courtesy that I expect in return.

I promise to encourage my partners to become familiar with my patients' medical condition and history to eliminate the need for asking questions already answered in the patients' medical record.

I promise to help my patient learn as much as possible with regard to the diagnosis.

I will welcome my patients' questions and provide clear answers to the best of my ability.

I will periodically remind my staff of the importance of courtesy and confidentiality.

I understand that this relationship may be terminated if my patient and I are unable to communicate effectively in order to ensure the provision of the best medical care.

_____
Patient's Signature

_____
Date   Physician's Signature

© 2003 by Margaret Smith Washington

Physicians who have achieved a partnership with their patients acknowledge the importance of effective communication. The doctor must encourage and reinforce patients' active participation in decision-making relative to their treatment plan. Patients must accept responsibility for learning about their illness so that they can share in the development of the treatment plan, and they must be responsible for monitoring their health status and noting significant changes on an ongoing basis.

A convenient tool to help patients monitor their health is a simple health log—a note pad, spiral notebook, or a bound journal. Its importance rests in the patient's dedication to recording information in it on a daily basis. A sample entry might read:

Monday (1/2/03) — Did my regular chores (made the bed, ran the sweeper); felt very tired by 2 p.m.-no pain, just tired.

Tuesday (1/3/03) — Slept late, right knee seems to be swollen, used ice bag, swelling went down.

This log should be shared with the physician on the next scheduled appointment. The information will assist in making a diagnosis and developing a treatment plan. The health log will also make the doctor aware that the patient has accepted responsibility for his/her care.

Physicians must make a concerted effort not to appear to be too busy to listen to patients who need to describe their "aches and pains" in a somewhat unfocused way. At the same time, the physician can take that opportunity to teach the patient how to become a more effective reporter and a more active partner in the relationship.

The patient's ultimate responsibility is to know his or her own medical history and to be prepared to share it with new physicians to whom a referral is made and with the staff in emergency rooms or urgent care centers. At a minimum, patients must know the medications they are taking and the reasons for taking them. They should also have a record of their hospitalizations and reasons for the hospitalizations. A medical history card, similar to the sample at the right, should be provided to all patients, and they should be encouraged to carry them at all times.

(front of card)

My Medical History		Name: _____	
Medicine	**How Often**	**Dose**	**Illness It Treats**

(back of card)

Hospitalization	Date	Reason

The card can be adapted to include space to record blood pressure or glucose readings, weight, or other data the patient may be required to monitor. Patients must take responsibility to remember to change the card when prescriptions are changed.

The Patient's Role

In a February, 2003, speech to a meeting of community leaders sponsored by the University of Pittsburgh Medical Center, Joycelyn Elders, MD, former U. S. Surgeon General, stressed the importance of patients moving "from health illiteracy to a status of health literacy." The ability of patients to do that, she said, "is dependent upon education, economics, environment, and a sense of empowerment." She urged health professionals to encourage patients to assume the responsibility for their care in a function she labeled "self management."

Patients must realize that this "self-management" of their diagnosis should be based on sound medical advice and not on observations of others with similar diagnoses. Patients who take an active role in their care ask questions, listen, and take responsibility for life-style changes. They must make a commitment to learn about their illness and to use their physicians as a resource in the learning process. Patients must understand the importance of communicating their fears and frustration in a manner that does not blame the doctor but rather seeks a clearer understanding, and they must assume responsibility for outcomes that result from their own inability or unwillingness to follow the prescribed regimen. In short, patients must commit to making their health a priority.

The Physician's Role

Physicians must embrace the concept of a viable partnership with patients that will allow and encourage patients to assume responsibility for their care. They must encourage patients to share information that might be personal but is essential in making the proper diagnosis. They must encourage patients to learn about their illness and welcome questions as a learning initiative rather than a challenge to their competence.

Physicians must help patients learn about access to the health care system and the appropriate use of the system, and patients must empower themselves to become an integral component of that system. Physicians and patients should work together to become more proactive with insurers and regulatory agencies and assure the availability of the necessary resources to provide and receive good patient care.

Physicians should ensure that their clerical staff members recognize the vulnerability of the patient and respond, rather that react, to patient "acting-out" behaviors. Both physicians and their clerical staff must be sensitive to patient scheduling and avoid long waits while encouraging patients to keep their scheduled appointment.

Preparing the Next Generation

Medical schools must integrate effective communication skills in all facets of the curriculum, and diversity training to achieve cultural competency should be a part of medical school and continuing education courses. Physicians who work in clinics and ambulatory care centers must take the time to learn the cultures of the communities that they serve to assure appropriate and acceptable behaviors.

South-Paul and Grumback in their research made the following observations and recommendations specifically for family practitioners, but the relevance to all practitioners is apparent:

The changing population mix, shifting gender balance, increasing proportion of elderly, and major socioeconomic trends and income disparities occurring in the United States today have shaped a practice environment that differs greatly from what faced family physicians 30 years ago. These changes necessitate a change in approach to training and practice. We recommend that family practice, as a specialty, consider adopting the following actions and attitudes:

First, advocate for a physician workforce that represents the population we serve. Major differences in health status, communication styles, and preferences for providers exist among our diverse patients. Both providers and patients are more likely to choose concordant therapeutic relationships. Family physicians may play a variety of roles in promoting a more racially and ethnically diverse medical profession, such as participating in medical school admissions committees and working with local school districts to enhance science education for disadvantaged students.

Second, it is important to recognize the disparity in numbers of minority providers compared to their representation in the population. Simultaneously we need to become more competent in caring for culturally diverse patients and more forthright about recognizing the legacy of racism that continues to influence the relationship between patients, physicians, and the health care system.

Third, there should be closer linkages between practices, clinics, and academic health centers and the communities they serve. These entities should become partners in improving the total health of the community.

Fourth, it is essential to better integrate minorities and women already in the profession into the framework of decision-making that promotes equity and success for those individuals. Attention must be directed and solutions found to breaking the glass ceiling that exists to the advancement of both groups.

Fifth, we must become more knowledgeable about the needs and strengths of our elderly patients and colleagues. As the number of elderly grows, skill in managing patients with chronic illness will become an ever more important element of family practice. And as the number of older physicians grows—a group with significant experience—they may be able to assist in addressing the needs of the underserved segments of the population.

Sixth, we should advocate for a system of universal health coverage in the United States so that the most basic component of health care justice is achieved. A publicly accountable, tax-financed system for all residents of the United States would be the most effective and equitable system.

Finally, we must appreciate the underlying social determinants of health and illness and work to reduce the socioeconomic disparities that are the breeding ground for premature morbidity and mortality.[7]

I endorse those recommendations as imperative if we are to strive for a more equitable health care delivery system. Physicians and patients must provide for each other opportunities to form a partnership of caring that recognizes their mutual value.

In practicing medicine, physicians must be guided both by the basic principles of biomedical ethics and by Beauchamp and Childress's four fundamental virtues: compassion, trustworthiness, discernment, and moral integrity.[2]

Communication is a powerful tool in clinical practice. As Wilson points out in the *British Journal of Nursing*, research has shown repeatedly that "good communication skills result in better clinical outcomes, a greater propensity to follow clinical recommendations and reduced risk of clinical negligence and complaints."[9]

There is no consensus among patients and doctors on the most appropriate model for the patient-physician relationship. Over the past century, the relationships have evolved mainly through trial and error. The emphasis has been on the part of the doctor to achieve the highest level of wellness for the patient while the patient seeks and expects wellness as soon as possible with a minimum of inconvenience. In my research and literature review, three models emerged that, I believe, address the importance of relevant relationships most clearly.

Models of Patient-Physician Relationships

Newman et al. trace the changes that have occurred over the last century. In the early 1900s, they point out, a physician's bedside manner compensated in part for the lack of scientific cures. With the growth of science and technology, interpersonal aspects were overshadowed. Gradually, however, there has been a renewed interest in "medicine as a social process." The authors note, "a physician can do as much harm to a patient with a slip of a word as with a slip of a knife."

They further define the three models of patient-physician relationships as follows:

It is the opinion of some people that the differential in power between the patient and physician is necessary to the steady course of medical care. The patient seeks information and technical assistance, and the physician formulates decisions, which the patient must accept. Though this seems appropriate in medical emergencies, this model, known as the **activity-passivity model**, has lost popularity in the treatment of chronic conditions such as rheumatoid arthritis. In this model, the physician actively treats the patient, but the patient is passive and has no control.

The **guidance-cooperation model** is the most prevalent in current medical practice. In this model, the physician recommends a treatment and the patient cooperates. This coincides with the "Doctor knows best" theory whereby the doctor is supportive and non-authoritarian, yet is responsible for choosing the appropriate treatment. The patient, having lesser power, is expected to follow the recommendation.

In the third model, the **mutual participation model**, the physician and patient share responsibility for making decisions and planning the course of treatment. The patient and physician are respectful of each other's expectations and values. Some have argued that this is the most appropriate model for chronic illnesses, where patients are responsible for implementing and determining its efficacy.[6]

Although all three models achieve varying degrees of success, my data validate the efficacy of the mutual participation model. In the 21st century, the impact of technology and the wide span of media exposure have produced a more sophisticated patient and, one would hope, physicians who welcome the active participation of patients. The role is new for both partners and requires a concerted effort from both to achieve the desired effect. The urgency of clearly articulated expectations and sensitivity to each other's values must be recognized and accepted. Where expectations are not realistic or achievable, the partners must seek reasonable alternatives.

Other Resources and Influences

The role of commercial insurance companies and governmental regulatory agencies in doctor-patient relationships emerges clearly from the surveys, focus groups, and interviews. These entities must enter into the dialogue with doctors and patients and seek strategies to address limited funding and inadequate resources or inappropriate use of resources. Partnerships must be formed with commitments on all sides to critically assess their ownership of slices of the conflict pie. Insurance carriers, for example, could provide physicians with formulary change notices in a more user-friendly medium (i.e., a laminated card for easy reference). Patients must be responsible for asking physicians to verify their insurance carrier's formulary prior to writing a new prescription, and they should be educated on the co-payment differential for generic vs. brand-name drugs. If each partner "owns" its contribution to the many problems, the result will be a modified health care system that will better serve patients, doctors, insurers, and regulators on a sounder basis.

Professional medical associations must acknowledge the crisis in communication between doctors and patients and take the necessary steps to address the problem. Some associations have already embarked on self-assessment beyond the expected clinical competence. Those associations that have not yet begun the internal critiques must step forward and embrace the urgency to revisit doctor/patient relationships in a time of technological advances and electronic information sharing.

The pent-up emotions witnessed at the patient focus groups are clear indications that health care providers (physicians, hospitals, and clinics) must provide regular opportunities for patients to share their concerns and frustrations. Most patients who "act out" or continue to be noncompliant are seeking assurance that someone is listening, caring, and willing to partner in resolving or modifying real or perceived barriers to care.

By the same token, the candor and frustration exhibited by physicians in their focus groups identified the need for ongoing peer dialogue outside of the day-to-day clinical environment. The clinical or treatment environment does not provide ample opportunities for physicians to share and learn from each other on matters outside of the normal clinical interactions.

Conclusion

Patients and physicians must begin or renew their relationship with a clear declaration of what they expect of each other in order to manage the illness of the patient. Time must be set aside to accomplish this task. Both partners must recognize that neither doctor nor patient possesses magical powers that allow them to read each other's mind. Both should assume nothing. They should ask—even when they think they know the answer. Redundancy in communication assures a more positive outcome.

The Challenge for Physicians

Physicians are ultimately responsible for teaching, learning, and partnering with their patients. They must see each patient encounter as an opportunity to broaden the patient's knowledge base with reference to the illness and to learn more about the patient as a person. Physicians must review with patients their medications and the purpose of each, acknowledge patient efforts to be compliant, and explore with patients the barriers that lead to non-compliance to arrive at a satisfactory resolution. Physicians must develop open dialogue with patients who have chronic illnesses to reinforce the importance of self-management. Those who treat acutely or chronically ill patients must recognize the patients' fear of the onset of illness and their lack of emotional and intellectual preparedness for its life-threatening potential.

More specifically, participants in our survey and focus groups offered the following suggestions for physicians:

- New technology is fine for diagnostic purposes, but doctors should invest in a human being to remind patients of appointments. One respondent said she was offended by an automated message that initially "sounded like the recorded pitch I receive periodically from a burial insurance telemarketer" and then proceeded to threaten all patients, regardless of their payment histories, that *"all co-payments and outstanding balances are due at the time of the appointment, or you will not be seen by the doctor."*

- Physicians should find time to discuss current concerns by *not* asking patients to repeat most of their medical history at the start of each appointment. Since doctors presumably learned to take good notes in medical school, they should use that training to maintain patients' charts and take a moment to review the notes before entering the examining room.

- Greeting patients by first name does not necessarily break the ice. It's not safe to assume that everybody is normally addressed by the first name on the chart or by a common nickname (e.g., Patty for Patricia or Walt for Walter). It's always safe to use the formal title (Mrs. _____ , Ms. _____, or Mr. _____)—particularly when the doctor is half the patient's age. Ditto for medical assistants, who may be young enough to be the patient's grandchild.

- Physicians should not be offended or condescending when patients refer to what they have read on the web or in medical encyclopedias. They're not questioning the professional's judgment; they're trying to understand their condition and treatment. Most patients are perfectly capable of learning; physicians should be grateful for their interest and the confidence they are expressing in the physician as a source of reliable information.

- As to information-sharing, patients want to know the results of those tests they take, particularly when "we" are tracking changes or effects of medications, and they want to hear them promptly—not a month after the blood is drawn and other changes are underway. And, yes, the "numbers" do mean something to the patient, especially when the provider takes the time to provide the normal range. Dropping the report in the mail is also acceptable, if there's no time to call. Not knowing test results can cause patient anxiety.

- And, finally, physicians should insist that the office staff is reasonable when they schedule appointments. Nobody is going to see five patients at 1 p.m., and patients who wait, often an hour or longer, for an over-scheduled doctor may become angry enough to look for a new referral.

The Challenge for Patients

Patients as a whole, and particularly those with long-term chronic illnesses, must develop the capacity to be attentive to their illness on a regular basis. To do so, they must develop an ongoing relationship with their doctor based on trust and mutual respect. Patients must make a commitment to learn about their illness and exhibit a willingness to partner with their physician by sharing information that will assist the doctor in an accurate diagnosis and treatment plan. Patients must learn to see the physician not only as the potential healer but also as a person who may share some frailties with their patients. Patients must assume responsibility for knowing their medications and their purposes, and they must strive for compliance with the treatment plan. When patients are not able to follow the plan, they must inform the physician and seek help in overcoming the barriers to care that cause the non-compliance.

Participants had the following suggestions for patients:

- Patients should learn how to describe their symptoms in a precise, meaningful way. Comments like "I'm feeling poorly" or "I'm doing all right, I guess" don't tell the doctor much about one's condition. "I'm very short of breath after climbing only a few stairs" or "I get a sharp pain just under my left rib cage whenever I take a deep breath" may be the first step towards a diagnosis.

- Keeping track of numbers (blood pressure for hypertensives, glucose levels for diabetics, hormone levels for various conditions, including hyper- and hypothyroidism, cholesterol and triglycerides, etc.) is very important. Patients should take note of any major changes in prescribed medications. If there is no significant change and the test results are stable, the change in dosage could be a clerical error. Patients should feel free to question the change. By the same token, patients should let each physician they see know about any chronic conditions they have, current medications they are taking, and any adverse reactions they have experienced with drugs.

- Patients must be aware of their rights. They have the right to all information in their medical records. They have the right to know the risks involved in any prescribed test or treatment, and they have the right to refuse treatment if they are told and understand the potential consequences of doing so. Physicians generally base their decisions on the patients' best interests, and patients are usually wise to follow their doctors' recommendations. Occasionally, however, physician-patient concerns, priorities, or beliefs come into conflict, and in such cases, the ultimate decision rests with the patient. In such cases, communication is especially important. Patients who are thinking about refusing treatment should discuss their concerns openly with the physician. There may be a compromise course of action that will satisfy both.

The ingredients of disrespect, mistrust, lack of cultural competency (failure to understand and accommodate racial, ethnic, and cultural differences), insensitivity, and poor communication of concerns combine to create a "conflict pie." Acknowledging the existence of the "pie" is the first step towards eliminating the conflict. Each partner (patient and doctor) must be willing to own responsibility for some slices in the pie (i.e., lack of availability, withholding information, mistrust, etc.) Once the ownership of the conflict slice is acknowledged, the owner must recognize how it contributes to the problem of communication and look for ways to eliminate or modify its impact. The ingredients serve as barriers to listening and hearing of patient and doctor concerns and frustrations. Mutual respect, open communication, and a willingness to accept responsibility for change will create a meaningful partnership for health—a partnership where each partner has an accepted, specific role and responsibility to make it work. For many physicians and patients, this will be difficult initially, but if each makes the commitment, the outcome will be satisfactory for both.

Ultimately, the patient will be heard and the doctor will listen; the doctor will be heard and the patient will listen.

References

1. Carroll L. (2000) *Alice's Adventures in Wonderland; Through the Looking-Glass.* New York: Penguin Group USA, Inc. (Signet Classic).

2. Gillant R. (1997) "Physicians' virtues and communicating with patients." *New Horizon* 5(1): 6-14.

3. LaCombe, M, ed. (1995) *On Being a Doctor.* Philadelphia: American College of Physicians.

4. *Holy Bible,* King James Version. (Corinthians 15:33). 1994. Grand Rapids, MI: Zondervan Publishing House.

5. Merriam-Webster. (1997) *Universal College Dictionary.* New York: Gramercy Books.

6. Newman S, Fitzpatrick R, Revenson T, Skevington, S, and Williams, G. (1996) *Understanding Rheumatoid Arthritis.* London: Routledge

7. South-Paul, JE, and Grumbach, K. (2000) "How does a changing country change family practices?" *Family Medicine* 278-285.

8. http://www.diversityresources.com/

9. Wilson, J. (1998) "Proactive risk management: effective communication." *British Journal of Nursing* (Aug. 13-Sep. 9); 7(15): 918-919.

10. Witzkin, H. "Doctor-patient communication. clinical implications of social scientific research." *JAMA* 1984 (Nov. 2);252(17): 2441-6.

Bibliography

1. Belasco JA. (1990) *Teaching the Elephant to Dance: Empowering Change in Your Organization.* New York: Penguin Books USA, Inc. (A Plume Book).

2. Cooper PL, Gallow J, Gonzales J, et al. (1999) Race, gender, and partnership in the patient -physician relationship. *JAMA* 1999; 282-583-9.

3. Hammer K. (1993) *And How Are We Feeling Today? The Impatient Patient's Hospital Survival Guide.* Chicago: NTC Contemporary Publishing Group (Contemporary Books).

4. Mechanic D. (1998) Public trust and initiatives for new health care partnerships: Effective communication between doctors and patients. *Milbank Quarterly* 76: 281-302.

5. Saha S, Komaromy M, Koepsell T, and Bindman A. (1999) Patient-physician racial concordance and the perceived quality and use of health care. *Arch Intern Med* 159: 997-1004.

6. Spector RE. (1991) *Cultural Diversity in Health and Illness*, 3rd ed. New Jersey: Appleton & Large.

7. Williams DR, Lavizzo-Mourey R, and Warren RC. (1994) The concept of race and health status in America. *Public Health Rep* 109 (1): 26-41

8. Medical College of Wisconsin. Medical schools working to improve doctors' communication skills. http://healthlink.mcw.edu/article/946506309.html